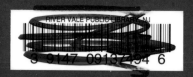

W9-AOY-130

JUICE IT, BLEND IT, LIVE IT

JUICE IT BLEND IT
LIVE IT

Over 50 Easy Recipes to Energize, Detox, and
Nourish Your Mind and Body

Jamie Graber

Founder of Gingersnap's Organic

Foreword by
Gabrielle Bernstein

New York Times bestselling author of *Miracles Now*

Skyhorse Publishing

Visit our website at www.skyhorsepublishing.com.

10 9 8 7 6 5 4 3 2 1

Library of Congress Cataloging-in-Publication Data is available on file.

Cover design by Brian Peterson
Cover photo credit: Noah Feck

Print ISBN: 978-1-63450-562-8
Ebook ISBN: 978-1-5107-0153-3

Printed in China

Table of Contents

SPIRIT · LOVE · ALERT

INSPIRE · ALIVE · BLISS · ENERGIZED

COMMUNITY · SMOOTHIES · INVIGORATE

CLEANSE · HEALTH · COMPASSION

ORGANIC

MANIFEST · CLEAN EATING · JOY

NUTRITION · DREAM · BREATHE

HAPPINESS · CREATE · SELF-CARE

VIBRANT · YOGA · JUICE

Acknowledgments

When they say it takes a village, this could not be more true. I have so many people to thank for helping get this book to you. To start, a huge thank-you to Gabby Bernstein, for telling me to say yes and for a beautiful foreword. To Christine Arroyo, for helping put the words on paper. To Anna Lownes, for tasting every recipe and giving me the thumbs-up or thumbs-down. To John Von Pamer, for the beautiful photos. To Theodora Sopko, for helping to lay each ingredient with such care. Lastly and most importantly, William Hickox, my loving and supportive husband, who not only styled the book, but inspires me every day.

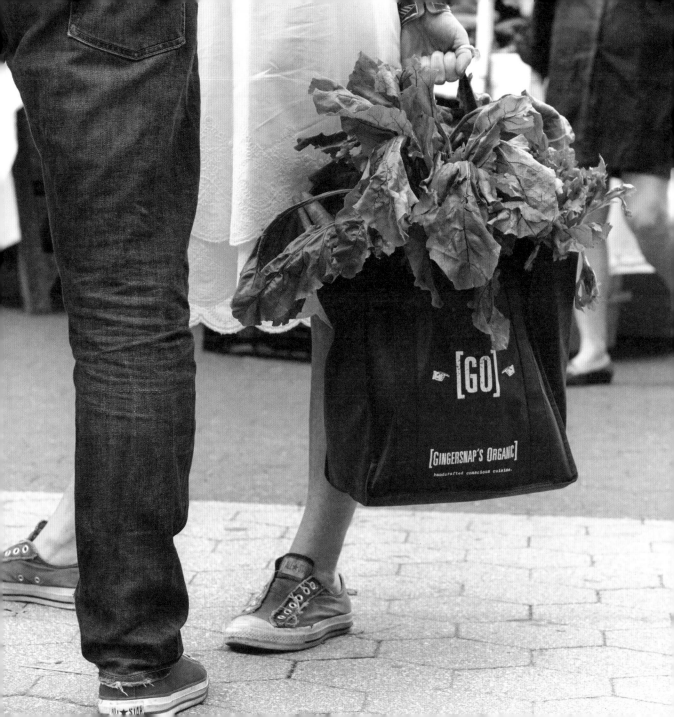

Foreword

One spring day, I was walking home and I noticed a new café had opened around the corner from my apartment. The chalkboard sign outside caught my eye. It had all my buzzwords: vegan, gluten free, cold-pressed juice, organic coffee. I thought, *OMG, heaven.* . . . I walked inside, and behind the counter was a young woman with fire-engine-red hair making a smoothie. I perused the menu and checked out the vibe. She looked at me and said, "We're not open for business yet, but can I help you?" I said, "Oh no! I was about to order one of your vegan, gluten-free donut holes." Then she said the magic words: "Take one; it's on me."

With one bite, I was hooked. Each day, I'd head to the new café, Gingersnap's Organic, to order my green juice and a donut hole. This became my routine. In time, this local juice joint became my favorite spot to hang, and Jamie, the red-tressed owner, became one of my best friends. Who knew that a vegan donut hole and a green juice could be the catalyst for a lifelong sisterhood?

Over the past few years, I've become a Gingersnap's Organic devotee. When I kicked sugar, I turned to Jamie to get me off donut holes and on smoothies. When I decided to cleanse, I asked her to create a special regimen for me. I became so obsessed with the Gingersnap's way that they actually named their [GO] Spirit Junkie cleanse after me! You know you're a regular when your name is on the menu.

The Gingersnap's way of eating and living has guided me through powerful healing transformations. Starting my day with a juice or a smoothie has offered a completely new way of living; it makes me feel connected and it's an important step in self-care. When you feed your body with whole greens, fruits, and all the natural ingredients Jamie has included in her recipes, you're nourishing your soul in an empowering, energizing way.

Cleansing and eating healthy foods has made a profound difference in my life, and now you can experience this same amazing gift. In her first book, *Juice It, Blend It, Live It*, Jamie gathers her miraculous recipes so that you can take your healing power back to the comfort of your home. What I love most about this book is that there are countless recipes that don't include fruit or any sweetener. I've been off sugar for the past two years, and Jamie's recipes have helped me kick the habit with grace and ease.

If you've been guided to pick up this book, then today is a very exciting day! You can take back your health, happiness, and energy one recipe at a time. And you'll have so much fun while you do it. There's nothing cooler than getting inspired to feel good. Let this book be your guide to shining from the inside out.

And if you're ever in New York City, stop by Gingersnap's Organic and treat yourself to a donut hole. You never know what will happen next. . . .

When you love your food, your food loves you.

Expect Miracles,
Gabrielle Bernstein

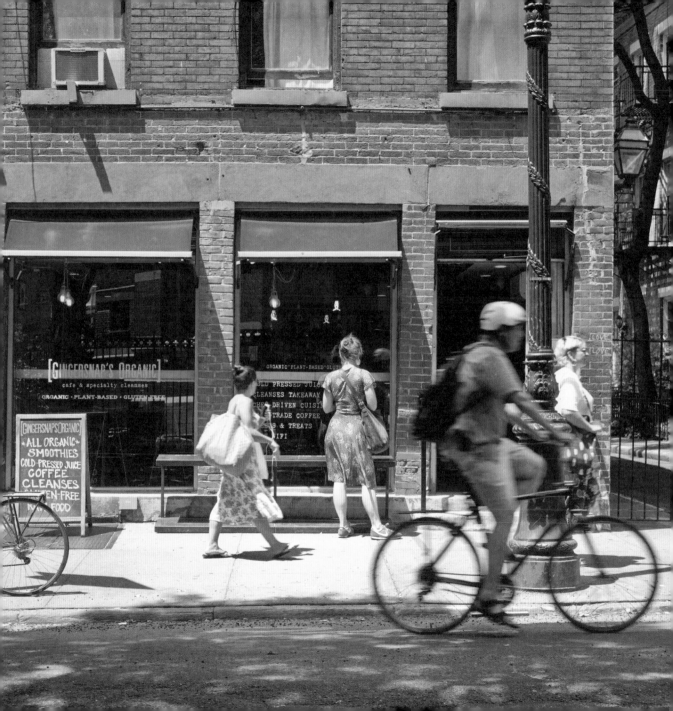

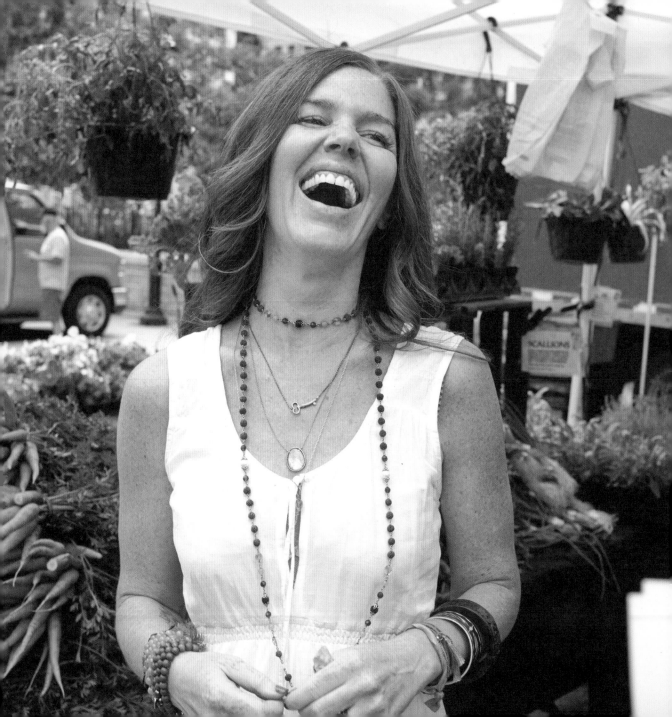

Introduction

"The journey of a thousand miles begins with a single step."—Lao-Tzu

We are constantly being bombarded with lists of what we should and shouldn't eat. There are hundreds of fad diets and rules for what to eat and when to eat it. With all of that constantly coming at us, when it comes to changing our diet, it can feel utterly paralyzing. I know about that firsthand because food had a similar effect on me in my late teens to early twenties. And ironically, in my struggle to control food, it ended up controlling me. I was a fashion-obsessed girl, reading every magazine I could get my hands on, thumbing through the pages of size-0 models, alongside the myriad ways to lose weight. I started to obsessively count my calories and my fat intake. Food became my enemy. With every bite of food, I feared I'd gain weight. After years of avoiding family dinners and outings to restaurants with friends, I woke up one day and knew there had to be another way. And so I began a journey to live a healthy and balanced life once and for all and to feel empowered about my food choices.

Juice It, Blend It, Live It is the result of my many years on this journey. My life is very different now, and I feel infinitely lighter and healthier now that I have removed the fear I always felt around food. I've replaced fear with joy and love in food. I am excited about food. I even married a carnivorous chef! We fell in love over food and the excitement we both get from a visit to the farmers' market.

When you are eating whole foods, the calorie and fat counting becomes unnecessary. You eat food the way nature intended it, and you find yourself full and satisfied instead of craving things that make you feel bloated and zapped of energy. But it's about balance. Now, if I know

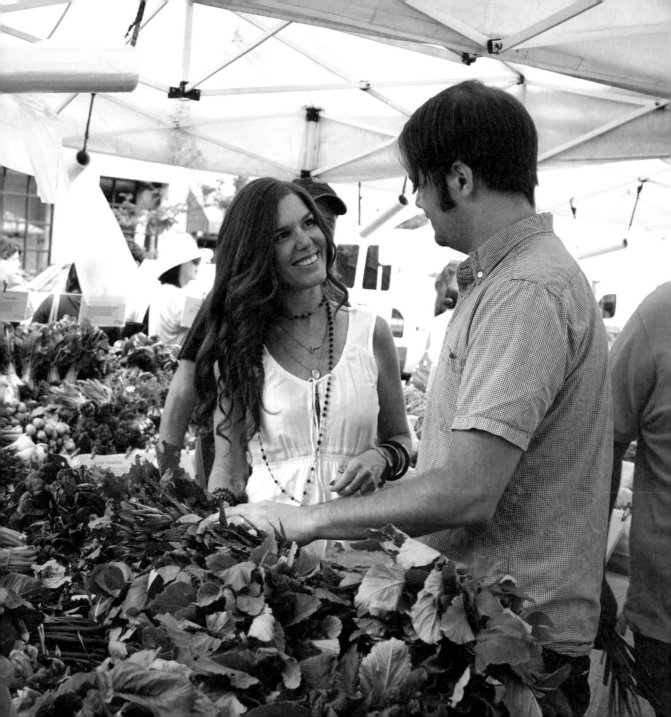

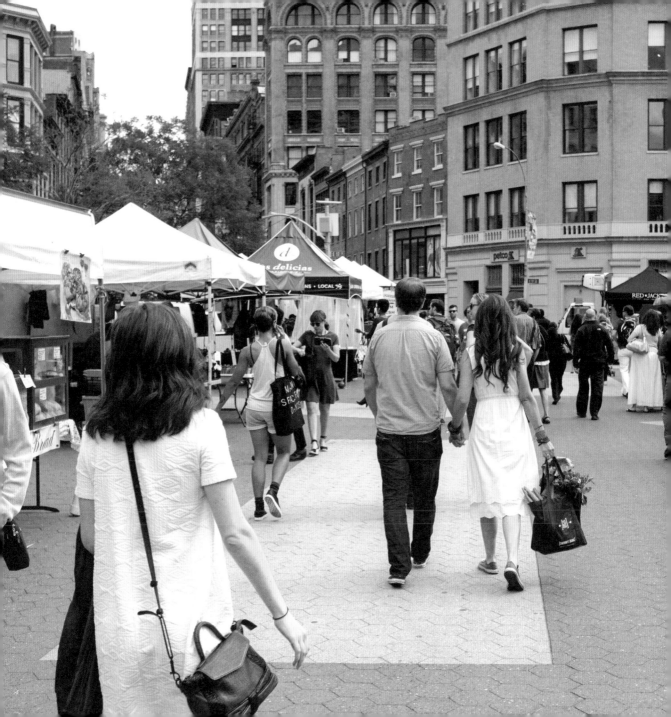

I will be having an indulgent, fancy dinner with my husband, I stick to just juice and smoothies the whole day. This way I go into the dinner feeling light but not starving. I hope you will find this book to be a guiding light into the change you're looking to make in your life. My goal is to leave you feeling empowered and energized after reading this book.

My journey to find balance, to be healthy, and enjoy food began with, quite simply, fruits and vegetables. Exploring the building blocks of food in its rawest form is an opportunity to really dive into the true nutrients of food and to think of food as what it is—a healthy and delicious source of fuel. I discovered that through adding juices and smoothies to my day, I felt lighter. My mind was clearer and I had more energy throughout the day. At the time, I lived near the ocean in Santa Monica, California, and I started to feel like I was in the flow of an amazing life/food balance that I'd never experienced before. I felt more connected to what food's true purpose is: to be a source of joy and energy to live the life of your dreams. The body is a temple that needs all the right nutrients and healthy ingredients to really function properly.

I began studying the nuts and bolts of juicing while working under Juliano Brotman, a pioneer in the raw food movement and owner of Juliano's Raw, a restaurant in Santa Monica, California. I left Juliano's Raw to become the manager for Euphoria Loves Rawvolution, a raw vegan restaurant and retail shop in Santa Monica. While there, I learned to create cleanses while also developing a partnership with YogaWorks, a popular yoga company, where I was able to teach clients how to balance their workout regimes with healthy diet and cleanse workshops. This inspired me to create a menu of raw juices, shakes, and soups for my clients.

In 2010, I left Los Angeles and moved back to New York City and took the ultimate leap by opening my own restaurant, which I playfully named "Gingersnap's Organic," after my own red hair. Gingersnap's Organic maintains my dedication to using high-quality, organic, sustainable, and environmentally friendly ingredients. Whether you live in a city or out in the middle of the woods, this book will give you the blueprint to live a healthy vibrant life. You'll learn a bit about different nutrients from different food sources; how to make delicious juices, smoothies, and nut milks; and different ways to incorporate these new recipes into your life. Whether you are looking to go on your own DIY cleanse or just adding a juice a day to your regular regime, I am confident that you'll feel lighter, more energized, and inspired to make the changes you've long been dreaming of.

I hope you will find this book to be a guiding light into the change you're looking to make in your life. My goal is to leave you feeling healthy and empowered.

So, let's begin!

How to Use This Book

"Take care of your body. It's the only place you have to live."—Jim Rohn

I've designed this book to be a jumping-off point for a healthy lifestyle. This book is for everyone—whether you are new to juicing or you've been doing it for years—you will find this book to be a great resource to go deeper into your journey. In the first part of this book, you will learn the different health benefits of the different ingredients in the book. All the juices, smoothies, and nut milks in here have been designed to bring you the most nutritional benefits in the tastiest way.

In addition to the recipes, I've also outlined cleanses and ways to combine certain juice and smoothie recipes. There will be beginner cleanses that might have more fruit, and others that are greens based. This is merely a guideline for how this can be a tool used to jump-start a journey into food choices that center around fruits and vegetables. While my recipes focus on plant-based foods, I've also outlined some add-ins, such as superfoods and spices to bring extra flavor, nutrition, or sweetness to your juice and smoothie.

Juicing and Blending—Why?

"The food you eat can be either the safest and most powerful form of medicine or the slowest form of poison."—Ann Wigmore

Most of us don't eat enough plant foods on our own. We fall short of the recommended daily amounts of fruits and vegetables in our diets. Juicing and blending smoothies are easy ways of introducing a variety of vegetables and fruits into your everyday diet. Juicing and blending makes it almost effortless to get your daily requirements of fruits and vegetables. Regardless of your lifestyle, most people agree more fruits and more vegetables is a healthier way to eat. That being said, sometimes it is difficult to include them in your everyday diet! That's where smoothies and juicing come in and make it much easier. For example, one green juice could have almost a head of kale in it and maybe even an apple, too, so in that alone, you are covered for half of your daily requirements. Again, the daily requirements are different for different people, but with juicing and smoothies, you are able to pack a lot of nutrients into one serving. It also satiates your body, filling it with vital nutrients so you are truly fueled to live the best, healthiest life possible.

I have chosen to focus on juicing and blending in this book because I think everyone can benefit by adding one of each to your day. It can change people's lives and health so drastically, and with this book, it makes it very simple. And when it comes to time and clean up, it takes less time than making eggs and bacon, plus your body will be thanking you! The section on nut and seed milks is also a great place for someone to start, especially if you are trying to remove dairy from your diet. The boxed nut and seed milks out there are filled with questionable ingredients and you'll be able to see how easy it can be to make your own at home!

JUICING

Juicing is a process that extracts water and nutrients from produce and discards the indigestible fiber.

Without the fiber, your digestive system doesn't have to work as hard to break down the food and absorb the nutrients. Juicing allows the nutrients to be immediately absorbed into the body. This allows your body to focus on healing itself on a deeper level because the energy your body would normally have taken to digest and break down the food is instead spent on rejuvenating. Juicing also adds the benefit of getting a larger and wider range of nutrition from different ingredients. When the fiber is removed, your body literally has more room for juice. And more juice means more nutrition. The less your body has to work, the more energy you have and the younger you feel and look. Juicing also makes the nutrients available to the body in much larger quantities than if you were to just eat the fruits and vegetables whole.

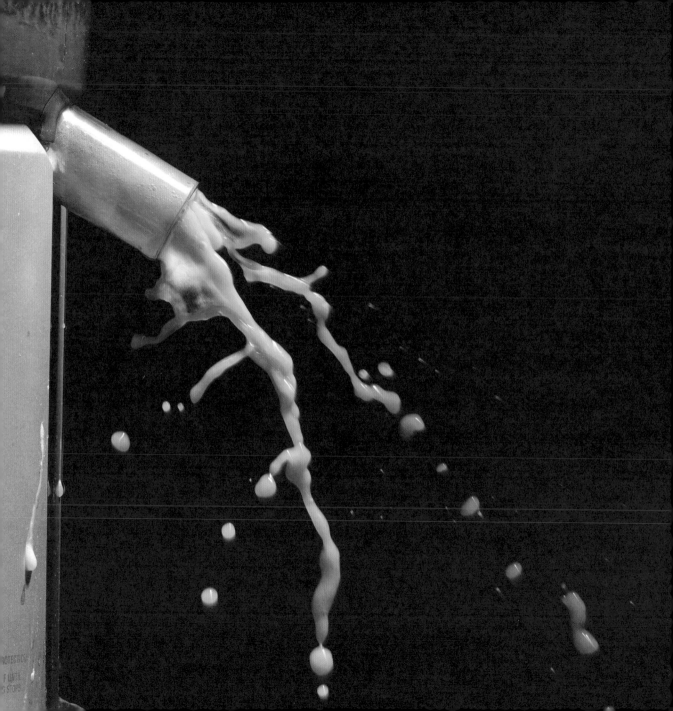

BLENDING

Smoothies typically consist of the entire fruit or vegetable, sometimes even the skin. The blending process helps to break down the fiber, making the fruit and vegetables easier to digest, and it also helps create a slow, even release of nutrients into the bloodstream, which keeps your body from avoiding the crash of blood sugar spikes. When blending smoothies, the fibers are still intact and the blade of the blender is being used like our teeth to break them down so the fiber is included with the other nutritious vitamins and minerals, making blending an excellent option that keeps the digestive system working well and helps smooth the colon and elimination process.

Smoothies are also more filling because of the fiber. More protein can go into the drink because, for example, you can put your chia seeds and superfoods into the mix. Don't be scared to put greens in your smoothies; they add important nutrients as well as enzymes that help digest the food. I recommend having more greens than fruits in your smoothie, especially if you're having a smoothie as a meal replacement. Try not to think of just sweet smoothies; savory ones are quite delicious, as well. Think of them as cold soups. You can even pour them into a bowl and eat them with a spoon!

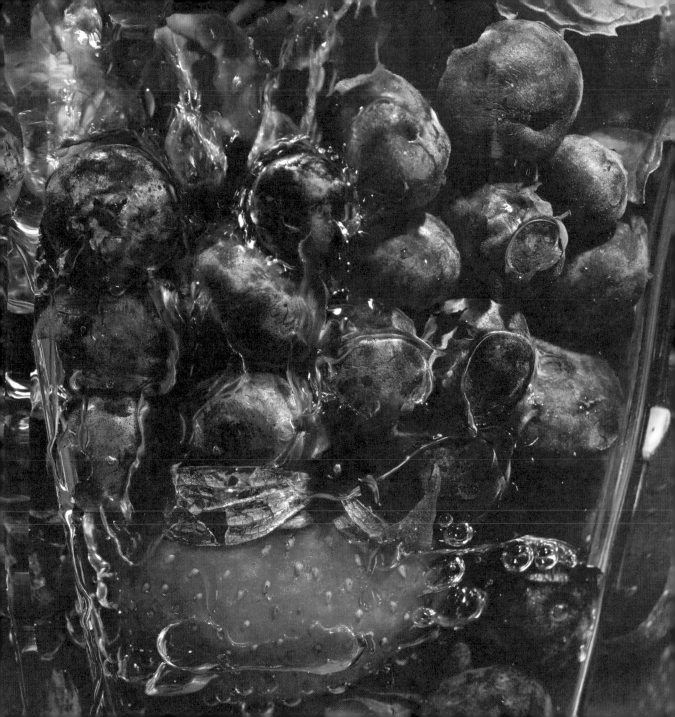

Substitutions

"Let food be thy medicine and medicine be thy food."—Hippocrates

If you are allergic, don't like the taste of an ingredient, or can't have certain ingredients included in this book, here's a list of suggestions for substitute options:

- Apples and pears are interchangeable. Other options are red grapes, cherries, blackberries, or blueberries.
- Arugula can be replaced by spinach, kale, or watercress.
- Instead of carrots, you can go with sweet potatoes or yams, pumpkin, or parsnip.
- Use basil or parsley in place of cilantro.
- Grapefruit can be replaced with clementines, oranges, tangerines, or blood oranges.

Fruits and Vegetables

"Eat food. Not too much. Mostly plants."—Michael Pollan

What can they do?

The basic building blocks to a healthy life are quite simply fruits and vegetables. My favorite greens to juice with are: kale, parsley, swiss chard, spinach, collard greens, and mint. My top fruits for juices and smoothies are: apple, avocado, bananas, berries, lemon, limes, mangos, oranges, pears, and pineapples. These are filled with nutrition. They also have great texture and create delicious drinks. They work well in balancing each other, as well as bringing out the best in each other.

Açai

This extraordinary berry's list of attributes includes a high level of antioxidants. Açai berries also contain excellent amounts of iron, calcium, fiber, and vitamin A. They also help defend the body against harmful free radicals. The health properties contained in açai berries may help prevent health problems such as arthritis, inflammation, and allergies.

Apples

Apples pack a powerful punch of vitamin C and B-complex vitamins. They also have good doses of calcium, potassium, and phosphorus.

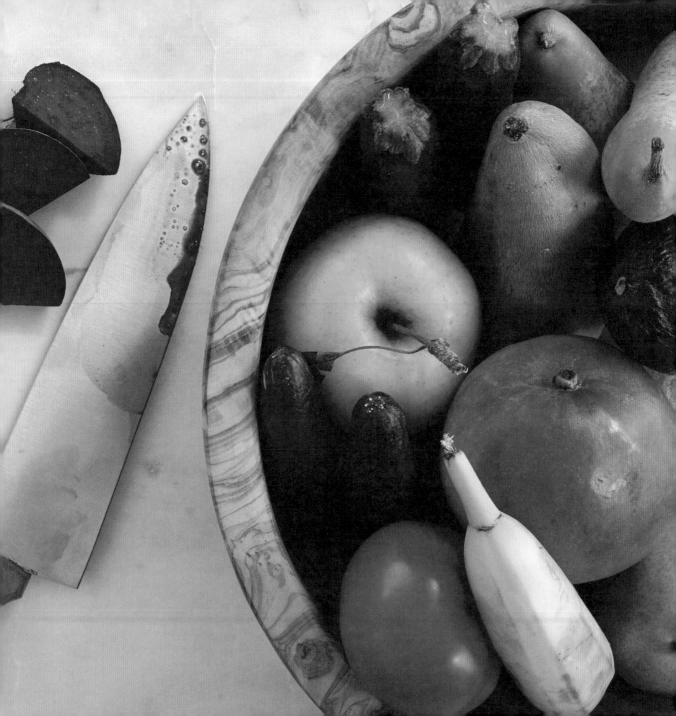

Avocados

Packed with monounsaturated fat and fatty acids, avocados can help lower LDL (bad cholesterol) levels while raising the amount of good cholesterol in your body. The healthy fats in avocados also promote the absorption of other carotenoids—especially beta-carotene and lycopene—essential for heart health.

Bananas

Bananas have potassium, which can lower your blood pressure, and they're also one of the best sources of a resistant starch. They're a healthy carb that fills you up and helps to boost your metabolism.

Beets

Beets are loaded with vitamins A, B1, B2, B6, and C. They are also an excellent source of calcium, magnesium, copper, phosphorus, sodium, and iron.

Blackberries

Blackberries are rich in polyphenols, the same family of antioxidants found in green tea, which may help prevent cardiovascular disease, cancers, and osteoporosis. Blackberries are also number one for fiber: one cup delivers one-third of your daily target of 25 to 35 grams a day.

Blueberries

Blueberries are full of phytonutrients that neutralize free radicals (agents that cause aging and cell damage). The antioxidants in these berries may also protect against cancer and reduce the effects of age-related conditions by keeping your mind sharp and preventing such diseases as Alzheimer's and dementia.

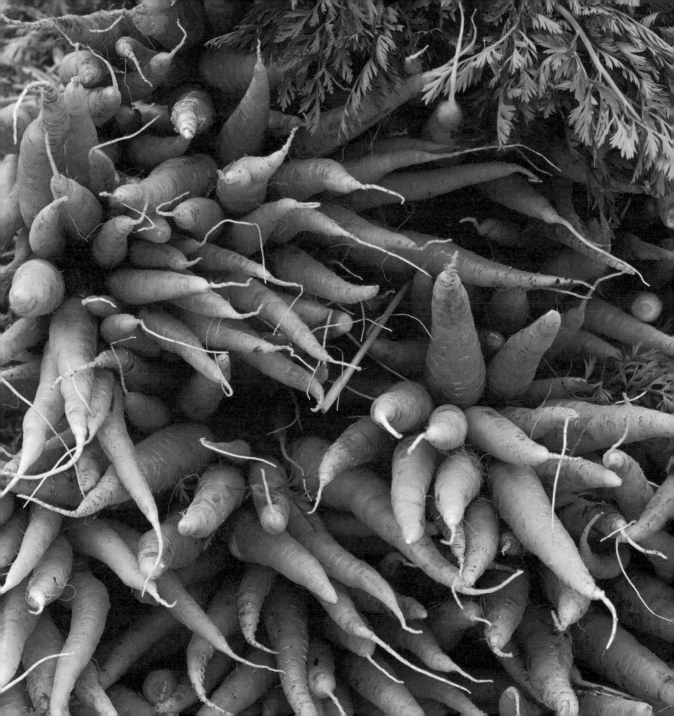

Burdock

Burdock contains the electrolyte potassium, which is an important component of cell and body fluids that helps control heart rate and blood pressure. This herb root also contains small quantities of many vital vitamins—including folic acid, riboflavin, pyridoxine, niacin, vitamin E, and vitamin C—essential for optimum health.

Cantaloupe

Cantaloupe has one of the highest sources of vitamin A of any fruit, while also being low in sodium, fat, and cholesterol. The excellent source of vitamin C it has defends the body against infection, and the potassium in it helps protect against stroke and coronary heart diseases.

Carrots

Carrots are an excellent natural blood sugar regulator. They have carotenoids, which actually helps balance blood sugar.

Celery

Celery leaves have high levels of vitamin A, and the stems have tons of vitamins B1, B2, B6, and C. Celery contains an abundant supply of potassium, folate, calcium, magnesium, iron, phosphorus, sodium, and plenty essential amino acids. Nutrients in the fiber are released during juicing, aiding bowel movements.

Chard

Chard contains vitamins K, A, and C, as well as magnesium, potassium, iron, and dietary fiber.

Citrus Fruits

All citrus, from limes to tangerines, are chock-full of vitamin C and fiber. It's the vitamin C that makes citrus an especially potent superfruit because this vitamin counters the effects of sun damage, regulates oil glands, and can even prevent age spots.

Lemon and lime peels contain about ten times more vitamins than lemon juice! They're also an excellent source of fiber, potassium, magnesium, calcium, folate, and beta carotene. Lemon peels improve bone health, too.

Collard Greens

Collards contain vitamin A and they're also rich in B vitamins, particularly niacin (B3), pyridoxine (B6), and riboflavin (B2), which are essential for overall body health. They also contain high levels of vitamin C and K.

Cucumber

Cucumber has an impressive amount of water that is naturally distilled, which makes it superior to ordinary water. Its skin contains a high percentage of vitamin A, so should not be peeled off.

Fennel

Fennel is very rich in vitamins A and C and many of the B vitamins. It is also an excellent dietary fiber.

Kale

The world is currently having a love affair with kale and for a good reason: kale contains a type of phytonutrient that appears to lessen the occurrence of a wide variety of cancers, including breast and ovarian.

Kiwi

Kiwi contains 273 percent of the daily recommended amount of vitamin C in every one-cup serving. It also contains vitamin A (great for skin, bone, and tooth development, and vision protection, including protection against macular degeneration), and vitamin E (twice the amount found in avocados, with nearly half the calories), along with potassium to balance the body's electrolytes and limit hypertension and high blood pressure. The copper in kiwi is especially good for children, supporting healthy development in infants, especially in the areas of bone growth and brain development. Copper is also important for the formation of healthy red blood cells and building immunity against disease.

Mango

Mango fruit is rich in prebiotic dietary fiber, vitamins, minerals, and polyphenolic flavonoid antioxidant compounds. It is an excellent source of vitamin A and flavonoids like beta-carotene, alpha-carotene, and beta-cryptoxanthin.

Parsnips

Parsnips are fiber rich, and research has shown there's a direct link between the intake of fiber-rich foods like parsnips and decreased chance of type 2 diabetes. A single serving of parsnips has nearly 7 grams of fiber, especially soluble fiber that aids in reducing cholesterol, as well as controlling blood sugar levels.

Pears

Pears contain good amounts of copper, iron, potassium, manganese, and magnesium, along with B vitamins like folates, riboflavin, and pyridoxine.

Pineapple

Pineapple contains bromelain, a digestive enzyme that helps break down food to reduce bloating.

Spinach

Spinach is very nutrient dense. It is low in calories, yet very high in vitamins, minerals, and other phytonutrients. It's an excellent source of vitamin K, vitamin A, magnesium, folate, manganese, iron, calcium, vitamin C, vitamin B2, potassium, and vitamin B6. It's also high in protein, phosphorus, vitamin E, zinc, dietary fiber, and copper.

Strawberries

Strawberries are bursting with vitamin C; just a cup full and you've already reached your recommended daily intake. They are also an excellent source of folic acid, which can help protect your heart.

Tomatoes

Maybe it's because I'm a redhead, but I've always loved a good tomato. You should love them too because they have lycopene, an antioxidant rarely found in other foods. Studies suggest that lycopene protects the skin against harmful UV rays, may prevent certain cancers, and lowers cholesterol. Plus, tomatoes contain high amounts of potassium, fiber, and vitamin C.

Watermelon

Watermelon contains good amounts of vitamin C as well as vitamin B6, which the body needs to help break down proteins.

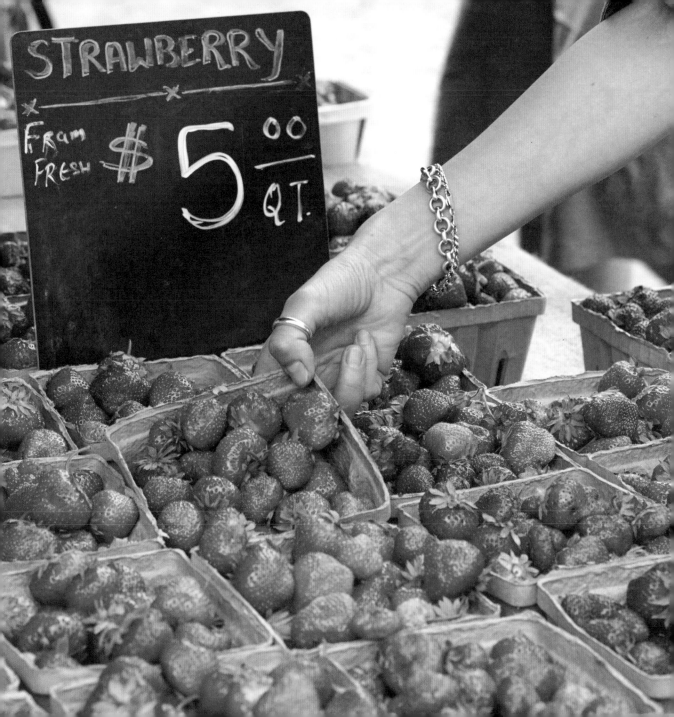

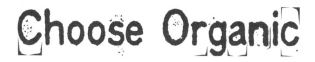

Choose Organic

Why Making the Organic Choice Is Important

Choosing organic is the first step in drastically reducing your exposure to harmful chemicals. Worldwide, six billion pounds of pesticides are applied to food crops every year. Organic growers are prohibited from using synthetic pesticides. Choosing fresh, organic ingredients not only lowers the amount of toxic pesticides in your body, but it can also drastically lower your levels of bisphenol-A phthalates. People don't realize these toxic ingredients can alter your body's chemistry. For example, bisphenol-A, when ingested, can alter your hormone levels.

Organic production also helps combat global warming. It absorbs carbon from the atmosphere rather than releasing it, as conventional farms do. Organic agriculture can bind 1,000 pounds of carbon from the atmosphere per acre. This is largely because organic production is based on building up healthy soil, which reduces water runoff and soil erosion, and provides better habitats for birds and fish in nearby waterways. Supporting organic farmers also reduces the amount of pesticides, such as atrazine, that enter our waterways and can harm aquatic life and end up in our drinking water. Farmers' markets and health-food stores are great places to buy your produce. Farmers' markets are great for local produce. Often, the produce at farmers' markets is not certified organic if it's from small farms. Speak to the farmer about their produce. Ask if they use chemicals or pesticides. They usually don't, but they cannot afford the paperwork to become certified organic. In these cases, support the small farmers and buy from them.

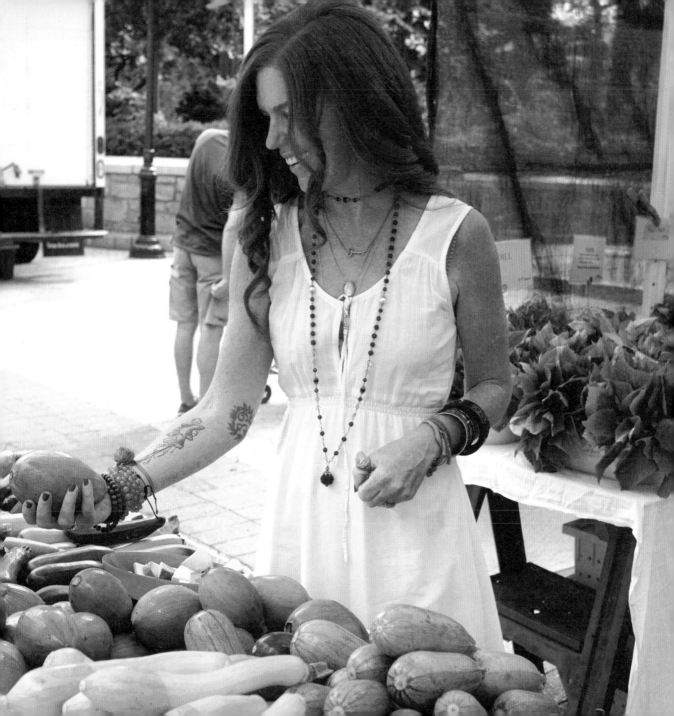

The Dirty Dozen

The Environmental Working Group (EWG) is a great resource for those looking to become empowered, conscious consumers. The following is their list of the twelve most pesticide-affected fruits and vegetables. Choosing organic for these fruits and vegetables is especially important. Please also consult their site as the list does fluctuate: http://www.ewg.org/foodnews/dirty_dozen_list.php.

- Peaches
- Kale
- Apples
- Sweet bell peppers
- Celery
- Nectarines
- Strawberries
- Cherries
- Pears
- Grapes
- Spinach

The Clean Fifteen

Although choosing organic is the best way to go, sometimes it's not always possible due to what's available or budgetary restrictions. The following is a list of fruits and vegetables that you don't have to buy organic if you're not able to. Again, please consult EWG's website for up-to-date changes as the list does fluctuate: http://www.ewg.org/foodnews/clean_fifteen_list.php.

- Avocados
- Sweet corn
- Pineapple
- Cabbage
- Sweet peas (frozen)
- Onions
- Asparagus
- Mangos
- Papayas
- Kiwi
- Grapefruits
- Eggplants
- Cantaloupes
- Cauliflower
- Sweet potatoes

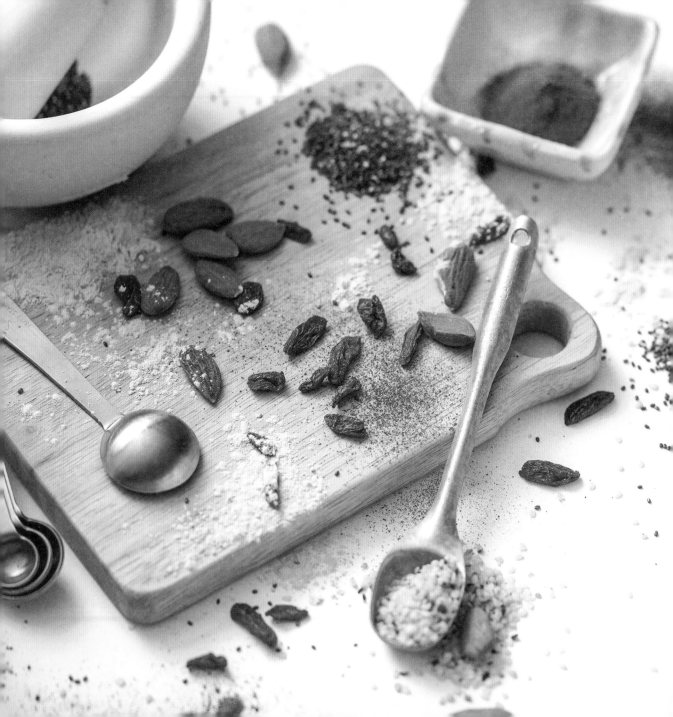

The Benefits of Nuts & Seeds

"The truly healthy alternative to that chip is not a fake chip; it's a carrot."—Mark Bittman

Nuts and seeds are a great source of protein and fiber. They can often give a creamy texture to your smoothies and are a great way to replace dairy. They taste so good, even kids love them!

Almonds

Almonds are high in monounsaturated fats, which can significantly lower risk of heart disease and lower cholesterol. In addition to healthy fats, almonds also have good doses of magnesium and potassium.

Brazil Nuts

Brazil nuts have selenium in them, which is a trace mineral essential to immune and thyroid function.

Coconut Flakes

Shredded coconut contains protein and fiber, which reduces your risk of constipation and hemorrhoids by encouraging proper digestion and regular bowel movements.

Pumpkin Seeds

Pumpkin seeds contain good doses of vitamin E and mineral antioxidants like zinc and manganese.

Sunflower Seeds

Sunflower seeds are rich in vitamin E and also have monounsaturated, saturated, and polyunsaturated fats that lower cholesterol and improve blood pressure.

Base Liquids

"If it came from a plant, eat it; if it was made in a plant, don't."—Michael Pollan

Having a base liquid, whether it's water or something else, is important to aid in the blending process. Here are my thoughts on options that I think work well in terms of texture and flavor.

While I do not believe in calorie counting, I do believe people can overconsume fruits and vegetables, especially when it comes to smoothies. And, to be honest, fruits and vegetables are so abundant in flavor, most can stand on their own in terms of taste! That being said, sometimes you want to be a little heavier and more decadent in your smoothies, so below are some options that can help to create a creamier and thicker smoothie:

Nut and seed milks offer a great creamy base for your smoothie. I've included recipes on how to make your own flavored milks. With all of these recipes, there's always the option to leave out the add-ins and drink them plain. They can also be used for smoothie bases or even with your granola or cereal in the morning. I do not suggest using the sweetened milks in any smoothie recipes. Also, I do not suggest using anything that comes in a box, that is shelf stable, and that has an expiration date of more than thirty days. If it does not have to be refrigerated, there is something in it that is clearly not natural. The same is true for anything that lasts more than thirty days. Coconut water is another great option. Cold water is a nice alternative when you want to make the smoothie lighter.

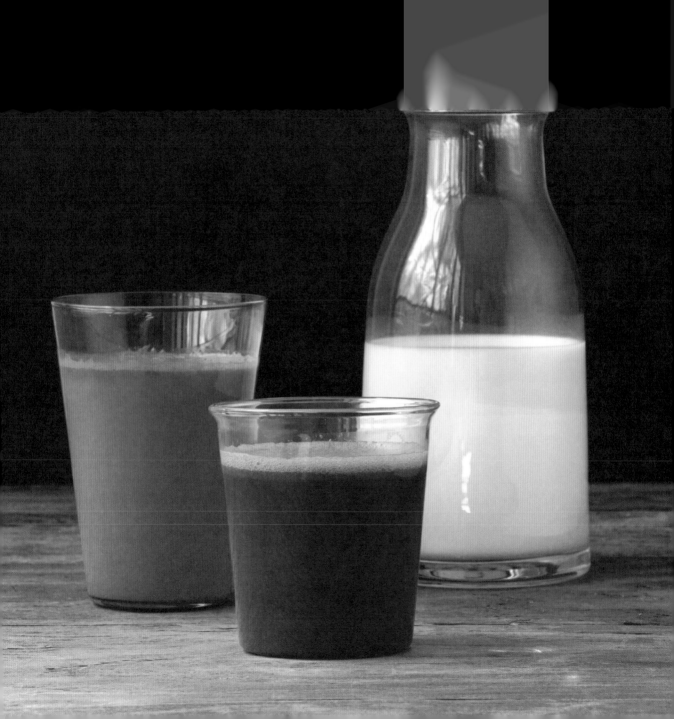

☞ Stay Hydrated

Hydration is always important, but especially with juicing and blending. I recommend drinking half your body weight in water. For example, if you're 100 pounds, you should drink 50 ounces of water. So whatever half your weight of water is in ounces is a good goal to try and keep. Often when we think we're hungry, we're actually just thirsty. After all, we are 90 percent water, which means staying hydrated is extra important. While plain filtered water is great, you can also make it a bit more exciting by making it "spa" water . . . Add things like slices of lemon, lime, mint . . . Get creative. . . .

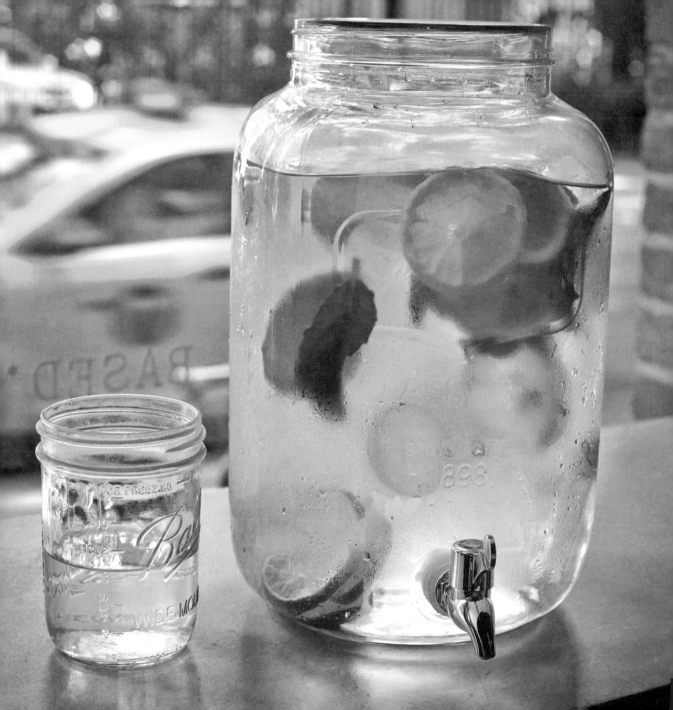

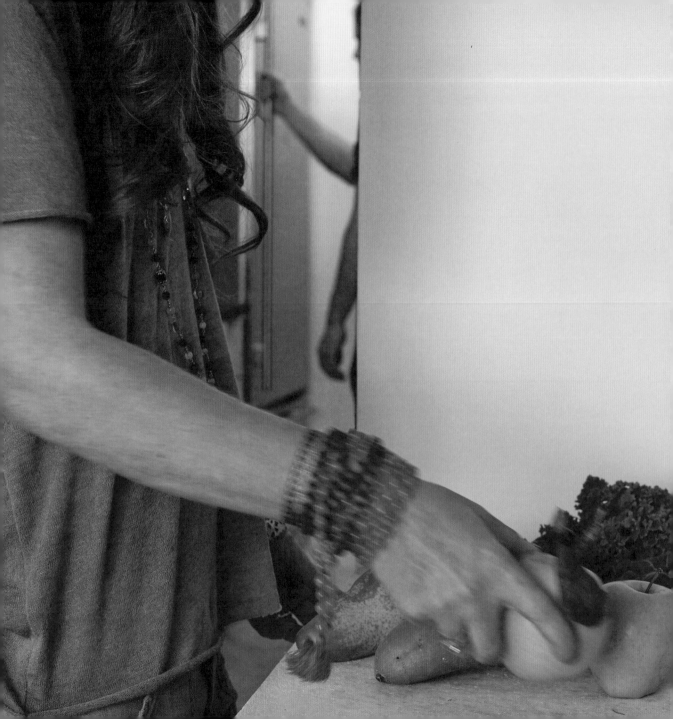

Caring for Your Fruits and Vegetables

Ripen: When it comes to avocados, tomatoes, mangoes, melons, apples, and pears, leave them on the countertop until they are ripe, and then put them in your fridge. Do not do this with citrus and berries, as they will rot. Bananas should be kept alone; they ripen quickly and can affect the fruits and vegetables around them.

Prewash: As you prepare for juicing, it's important not to prewash your vegetables. Wait until right before you're about to use them, because if you wash them too early, it cuts their shelf time in half. Also, do not precut them—the fruits and vegetables will start to oxidize and lose their nutritional value.

Storage: If they are tied together, remove the ties and if you see any decaying parts, remove those from the vegetable. Do not cram your vegetables together, as they will go bad quicker. Give them space to breathe. If you are keeping them in a bag, make sure there are small holes so they can get air. A good rule of thumb is not to keep fruits and vegetables together.

Freeze: For smoothies, another easy prep trick you can do beforehand is freezing your nut milk in ice cube trays. I also like for the fruit to be frozen because it gives a nice texture to the smoothie and helps prevent waste. But greens, herbs, and softer fruits, like berries and cherries, should be purchased more regularly at the local farmers' market or health-food store. Larger grocery stores are also starting to carry more organic produce so there are more and more options available.

If you are going to choose juice that's already made, I recommend staying away from pasteurized juices and HPP processed juices. The best option is a cold-pressed juice that hasn't gone through HPP. HPP stands for high-pressured processing. What that means is that the juice has gone through a pasteurization process that extends its shelf life for up to a month. HPP is not technically fresh when it has a shelf life of a month. The process also sterilizes. It's technically processing the juice, making it no longer fresh.

Storing Juices & Smoothies

When it comes to storing juices, some storage is going to depend on the juicer you're using.

If you're going to save the leftover juice, use a darker glass color for storage and then put it in an airtight container and place it in the back of the refrigerator. You can also get creative and freeze the juice in ice cube trays. Then, when you are making smoothies, you can add a little extra nutrition by throwing in one or two! With smoothies, the same process applies, but your smoothie may settle and change consistency when you store it in the refrigerator.

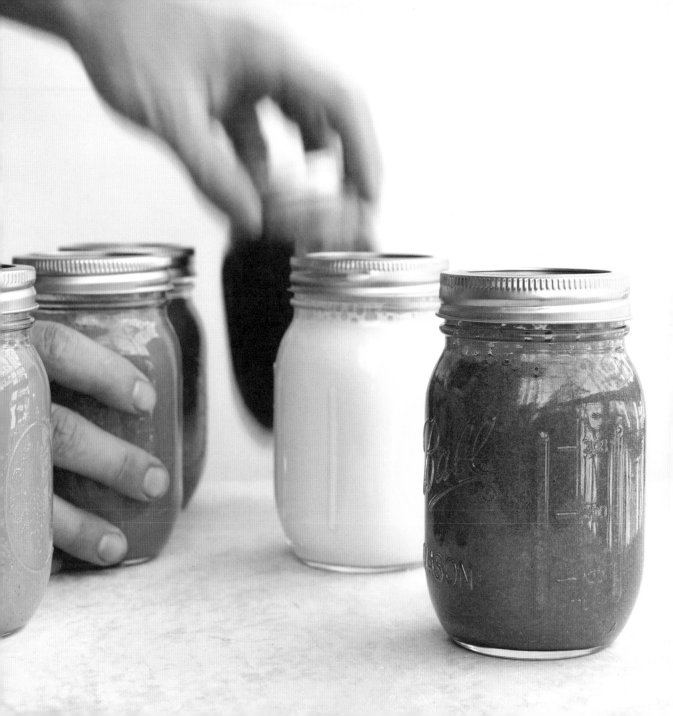

Superfoods

"The best strategy we have is to just add the good stuff! Eventually it's going to crowd out the bad stuff."—David Wolfe

What are they?

Superfoods are nutrient-rich foods that pack an extra powerful punch. They go the distance when it comes to giving your body large doses of antioxidants, polyphenols, vitamins, and minerals. I've called out a few of my favorites. While I don't use all of these in the recipes in this book, they are great to add to smoothies. You can find many of them in your local health-food store or online.

Cacao

Cacao is loaded with flavonoids, which are chemicals found naturally in plants that help fight a variety of conditions including diabetes and heart disease. Cacao also has flavonols, which can relax your blood vessels and thin your blood, naturally lowering your blood pressure numbers.

Chia Seeds

They're rich in antioxidants, vitamins, minerals, and fiber, and this super seed also contains 500 percent more calcium than milk and the same amount of omega-3s as wild salmon. Another side benefit of chia is its appetite-suppressing quality, helping you feel full and making them an ideal part of a weight-loss regimen.

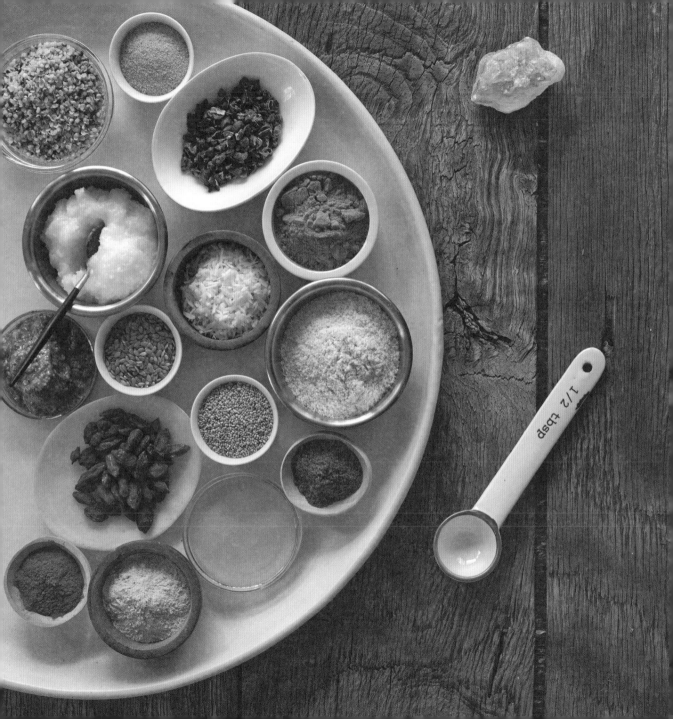

Coconut Oil

Coconut oil is another magical superfood that can boost thyroid function as well as aid with digestion. It reduces cholesterol and keeps weight balanced. Coconut oil is quickly digested and goes straight from your gut to your liver. Because it's one of the good oils that's mostly digested, it doesn't turn to fat, but instead quickly converts to energy. Coconut oil is also great on the skin for moisturizing and combating eczema.

Flaxseeds

Flaxseeds are a great source of high omega-3 fatty acids. Flaxseeds also have lignans, which are fiber-like compounds that provide antioxidant protection. They can also help in preventing excessive inflammation and protecting blood vessels. Their antioxidant and anti-inflammatory benefits also make them a great candidate for cancer prevention—particularly that of breast cancer, prostate cancer, and colon cancer.

Goji Berries

Goji berries are the most nutritionally dense fruit on Earth. They contain all essential amino acids and also have the highest concentration of protein of any fruit. They are loaded with vitamin C, contain more carotenoids than any other food, have twenty-one trace minerals, and are high in fiber. Boasting fifteen times the amount of iron found in spinach, as well as calcium, zinc, selenium, and many other important trace minerals, there is no doubt that the humble goji berry is a nutritional powerhouse.

Hemp Seeds

Hemp seeds are a complete protein. They have the most concentrated balance of proteins, essential fats, vitamins, and enzymes combined with a relative absence of sugar, starches, and saturated fats. Hemp seeds are one of nature's perfect foods—a true superfood. Raw hemp provides a broad spectrum of health benefits: weight loss, increased and sustained energy, lowered cholesterol and blood pressure, reduced inflammation, improvement in circulation and immune system, as well as natural blood sugar control.

Lucuma

Lucuma is high in carotene, which is an antioxidant that rejuvenates and reduces the effects of aging. It's also great for eyesight. It's high in iron, niacin, and fiber. It's also anti-inflammatory, with an anti-aging and skin repair effect on human skin. Using lucuma in place of sugar means you reduce your chance of suffering from all the health problems that processed sugar causes.

Maca

Maca is rich in vitamins B, C, and E. It provides plenty of calcium, zinc, iron, magnesium, phosphorous, and amino acids. Maca balances hormones and increases fertility. It's also known for increasing stamina and energy. Many athletes take maca for peak performance. If you find yourself feeling tired most of the time, experiment with maca to see if it helps. Just a small amount could be exactly what you need for a boost. Maca is also an excellent mood balancer and has been credited with relieving symptoms of anxiety and stress.

Tocotrienols

It's a highly potent source of vitamin E, which is great for your hair and skin. It's great to add to any smoothie or milk as it creates that custardy, deliciously creamy texture.

Turmeric

This antioxidant, antiseptic, and anti-inflammatory spice is a prominent medicinal tool in Ayurveda, the ancient medical tradition that began in India, where turmeric is widely used. Curcumin, the compound that gives turmeric its deep golden color, may protect against cancer and Alzheimer's. It also improves circulation and prevents blood clotting.

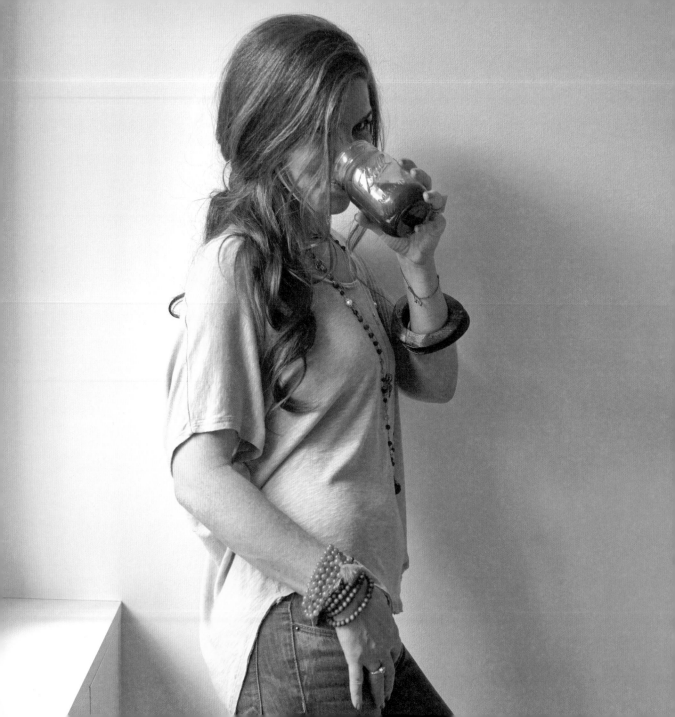

Medicinal Mushrooms

The following mushrooms are great for making teas that act as a supplement to your juicing and smoothie efforts. You can find these as whole, dried mushrooms or in powder form.

Chaga

Chaga mushrooms, when consumed on a regular basis, can slow aging, improve health, and provide anti-aging benefits. And because of immuno stimulation, Chaga mushrooms also fight against cancerous growths and cancer cells. The presence of betulinic acid in Chaga mushrooms inhibits the growth of tumors, and kills off tumor tissues, and tumor cells. So if you suffer from tumors, it is beneficial to consume Chaga mushrooms. Chaga mushrooms are your safest bet when it comes to creating general feelings of well-being and delaying the signs of aging.

Cordyceps

Cordyceps is a fungus that's used to treat coughs, chronic bronchitis, respiratory disorders, high cholesterol, dizziness, and weakness. It's also used for strengthening the immune system, improving athletic performance, reducing the effects of aging, promoting longer life, and improving liver function in people with hepatitis B. It can also be used as a stimulant to increase energy and stamina and reduce fatigue.

Reishi

Reishi is another amazing mushroom credited with boosting the immune system. It helps in lowering blood pressure and cholesterol, chronic fatigue syndrome, and reducing stress.

Herbs

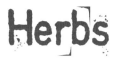

Herbs are powerful healing agents, and because they pack an extra powerful punch, they can take an ordinary juice and make it extraordinary.

Basil

Basil is considered one of the healthiest herbs. It's best when fresh. Its impressive list of nutrients includes vitamin K (essential for blood clotting) and vitamin C. Just 2 tablespoons of basil provides 29 percent of the daily recommended value.

Cilantro

Cilantro is a powerful, natural cleansing agent. The chemical compounds in cilantro bind to toxic metals and loosen them from the tissue. Many people suffering from mercury exposure report a reduction in the often-cited feeling of disorientation after consuming large and regular amounts of cilantro over an extended period of time.

Mint

Mint is a great palate cleanser and it promotes digestion. It also soothes stomachs in cases of indigestion or inflammation. Mint is a natural stimulant, and the smell alone can be enough to charge your batteries and get your brain functioning on a high level.

Parsley

This tiny-leaf plant is rich with chlorophyll, vitamins A, B, C, and K, folate, and iron. It has high beneficial mineral contents like calcium, magnesium, manganese, phosphorus, potassium, sodium, vanadium, and zinc.

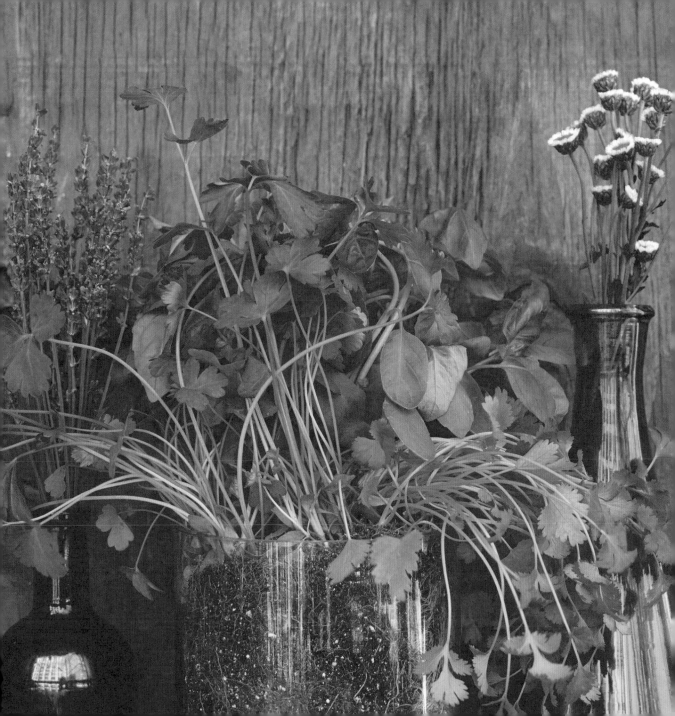

The Tools You'll Need

What Juicers Work Best

When people think of juicing, they think it's messy, complicated, and takes too much time. However, it doesn't have to be that way, and the first step toward making juicing an effortless part of your daily routine is having the right equipment. Luckily, there are lots of juicer options on the market and it's important to find the one that best suits your needs.

Some juicers will save you money, others will save you time, and some will even extend the shelf life of the juice. Of all the juicers I've test driven, these are my favorite ones.

But first, I'll explain the difference between juicers you'll find on the market so you can make the best decision that suits your needs.

Centrifugal juicers use a fast-spinning grater. The juice gets spun through a strainer and out the spout, while the pulp ends up in a catch basket. The good news is that it's easy to clean and use, it juices fast, takes up less counter space, is less expensive, and juices both fibrous veggies and larger pieces of produce well because it has a bigger chute. Some of the cons are that it's noisier and the juice it makes has a shorter shelf life of just 20 to 30 minutes. I used a centrifugal juicer to create the recipes in this book.

Centrifugal juicers I recommend are: Breville Juice Fountain Multi-Speed, Breville Juice Fountain Compact, Omega 4000 Juicer, Jack Lalanne Power Juicer Pro, and Black & Decker Fruit & Vegetable Juice Extractor.

Masticating juicers use one slow-turning screw-shaped gear that squeezes the juice through a stainless-steel screen. The perk is that it extracts more juice, and with a higher nutritional value, there's less foam and a longer fridge life (24 to 48 hours). Most of these models also juice wheatgrass and easily make nut butters, ice cream, veggie pâtés, and more. The cons are that it has a smaller chute, which means you have to chop the fruits and veggies into smaller pieces, it's a little more difficult to assemble, and there's a slightly higher price tag. You will also have to strain your juice if you use this type of a juicer.

Masticating juicers I like include: Breville Fountain Crush Masticating Slow Juicer, Hurom Masticating Slow Juicer, Omega Nutrition Juicer, Omega Vert, and Champion Household Juicer.

Twin gear juicers work at even lower speeds, slowly squishing the fruits and veggies between two gears. The juice stays fresh longer (about 72 hours), there's a higher juice yield, and it's also versatile—it easily juices wheatgrass and makes nut butters, ice cream, veggie pâtés, and more. It's also very quiet. The cons are that you have to chop the veggies into smaller pieces because again the chute is smaller, it's a larger and heavier machine, and it's slightly more expensive.

Twin gear juicers I like include: Super Angel 5500, Samson Green Power Twin Gear, and Green Star Elite Jumbo Twin Gear Juice Extractor.

The Norwalk Hydraulic Press is the best juicer out there. It literally presses the juice out of fruits and veggies including tough-to-juice grasses like wheatgrass. This juicer makes 50 to 100 percent more juice and contains three to five times more vitamins and minerals than juice pressed from other machines. The juice stays fresh for about three days. The cons are that it's a large and heavy machine and it's quite expensive. It also is very time-consuming.

Wheatgrass juicers work by slowly squeezing and pressing juice out of the tough wheatgrass fibers. Wheatgrass juicers come in either hand-crank or electric versions. Some wheatgrass juicers also juice certain leafy greens, vegetables, and fruits.

The more popular wheatgrass juicers are: Lexen Healthy Juicer, Z-Star Manual Juicer, Chefs Star Manual Hand Crank, Handy Pantry HJ Hurricane.

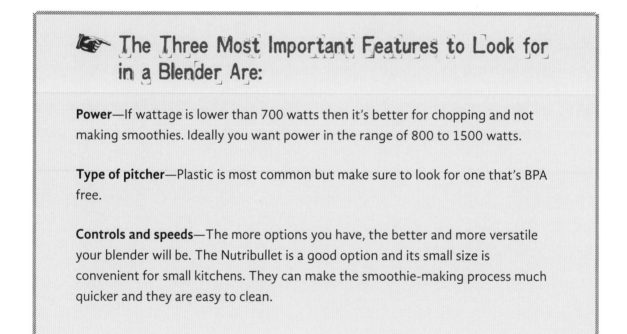

☞ The Three Most Important Features to Look for in a Blender Are:

Power—If wattage is lower than 700 watts then it's better for chopping and not making smoothies. Ideally you want power in the range of 800 to 1500 watts.

Type of pitcher—Plastic is most common but make sure to look for one that's BPA free.

Controls and speeds—The more options you have, the better and more versatile your blender will be. The Nutribullet is a good option and its small size is convenient for small kitchens. They can make the smoothie-making process much quicker and they are easy to clean.

How Your Soul Gets Fed

When you take care of yourself, your life gets better, you take more pride in what you do, and you feel better. What I love about eating clean is that it brings an overarching feeling of gratitude for your food and for your body. When I'm in the process of making smoothies and juices, I always remind myself to be grateful and to feel gratitude for the nutrition these ingredients are bringing me. In the cleansing and eating-clean process, it's important to honor yourself, because every choice you make brings you more into the flow. Soon you will come to see that food is fuel and, while this food is delicious, it's also fueling you and giving you the energy you need to live an amazingly inspired and energetic life!

But, it is not just about the food you put in; you want to fuel yourself with your surroundings, as well. That can mean surrounding yourself with friends who are positive and encouraging, listening to music that gets you wanting to dance, or reading books that make you feel empowered. For me, I start every morning with a lesson from the book *Course in Miracles* followed by a cuddle session with my husband. It's a great way to get grounded so I know that I can take on anything that comes my way with grace and ease. For some, the most important meal is actually their meditation, their yoga class, or even a journaling session . . . whatever it is that makes your heart sing, start your day from a place of gratefulness and joy.

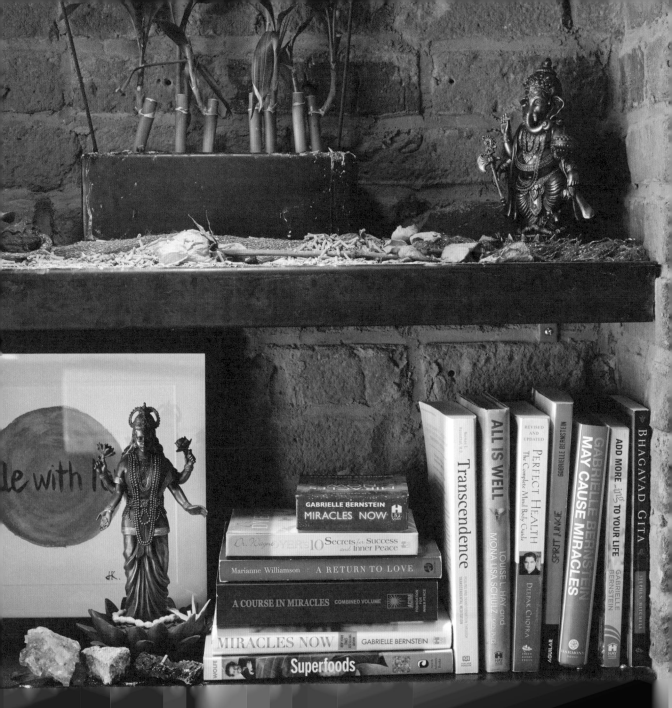

"It is essential to our well-being, and to our lives, that we play and enjoy life. Every single day, do something that makes your heart sing."—Marcia Wieder

What makes your heart sing?

_____

_____

_____

_____

_____

_____

_____

_____

_____

_____

_____

_____

_____

_____

_____

Go Lightly with Sugar and Fat

"Your health is what you make of it. Everything you do and think either adds to the vitality, energy, and spirit you possess or takes away from it."—Ann Wigmore

In the recipes in this book, I've been very careful not to use too much sugar because sugar, even sugar from natural sources, can significantly compromise your health goals. Fat doesn't make you gain weight, sugar does. Many health experts agree that sugar consumption may be the largest factor underlying obesity and chronic disease in America. Your body metabolizes fructose much differently from glucose; the entire burden of metabolizing fructose falls on your liver, where excess fructose is quickly converted into fat, which explains the weight gain and abdominal obesity many people struggle with.

I've also gone light on the fruits in these recipes, but if you want it sweeter, feel free to add a bit more fruit, though I recommend going as thin on the fruit as possible since the sugar in fruits is something to be wary of.

I am not suggesting you avoid fruit all together, but just be mindful of overdoing it. Start with less, and if you must, then add a little more. You will also notice I do not add sweeteners to any of the recipes because I believe the fruits, vegetables, and seeds can speak for themselves. But if you really want to add in a sweetener, my suggestions would be to use either coconut palm sugar or honey, and for nonglycemic sweeteners, try mesquite, xylitol, or stevia.

You'll notice that there aren't any oils or added fats in these recipes except for coconut oil. That's because the vegetables speak for themselves, and even with a savory soup, there's enough flavor to make it absolutely delicious. If you are looking to make it a little heavier and fuller, you can add a teaspoon of olive oil or ¼ to ½ of an avocado. This will make soups or smoothies a bit creamier.

👉 How to Add Superfoods and Sweeteners

I haven't included any superfoods in the following smoothie recipes, but if you'd like to add them in, then below are my recommendations. Here are some helpful tips on how much to use and how to prepare the superfoods for the most benefit.

Cacao—can be added into any of the smoothies or milks. It's unsweetened and bitter so you might want to counterbalance it with honey or palm sugar, but be mindful of how much honey or palm sugar you use.

Chia Seeds—make sure you soak them before (I'd recommend soaking them overnight) then add a tablespoon into any recipe and they'll act as a thickener without changing the taste.

Flaxseeds—a tablespoon can be added to the smoothies.

Goji Berries—add only a tablespoon to the smoothies or nut milks. The best option is to soak them overnight before using.

Hemp Seeds—a tablespoon can be added to any smoothies or milks.

Lucuma—is a nice sweetener for any of the smoothies without being high glycemic and it creates a nice texture.

Maca—great for smoothies and milks, but use only a quarter of a teaspoon.

Sweeteners—I made a point not to add any artificial sweetener in the recipes because fruits and vegetables speak for themselves, but if you are going to add a sweetener then I recommend coconut palm sugar, honey, and for nonglycemic sweeteners, mesquite, xylitol, or stevia.

Turmeric—you can buy it in powder form and I suggest adding only a small amount or a pinch.

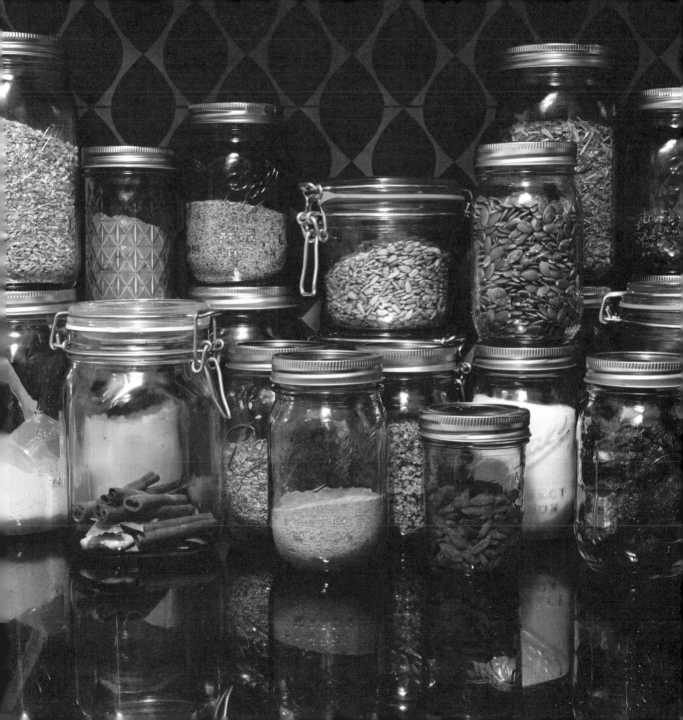

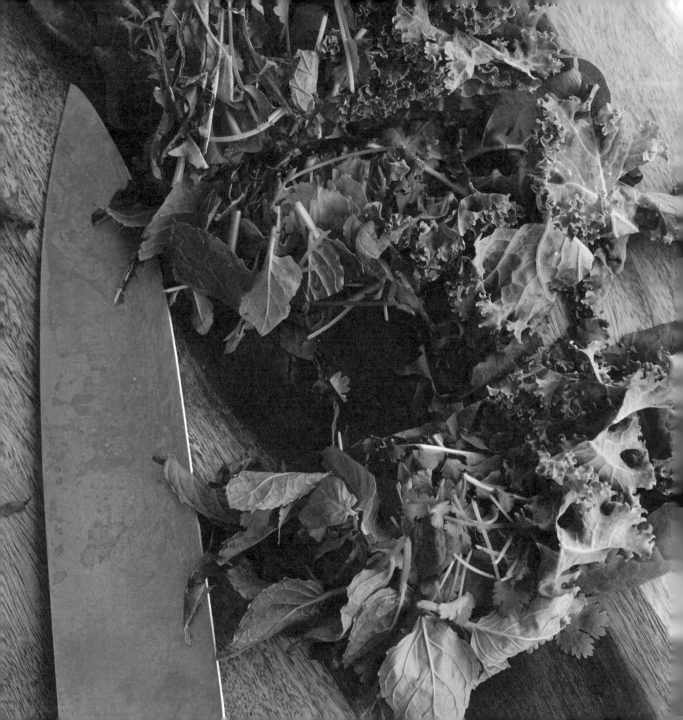

Juicing Tips

Before Juicing—*Please look at the below information before making any of the juice recipes. It will help you get the most out of all your fruits and vegetables!*

1. Always make sure your juicer is on before you put anything in it.
2. Wash everything thoroughly.
3. Lemon and limes are even better for you with the skin on, so you can keep it on if you like. If it is too bitter, leave half on.
4. Peel grapefruits and oranges, but leave the pith on.
5. It's also great if you leave the skin on your ginger.
6. 1 handful = 1 packed cup
7. Pack small leafy items with other ingredients to give you the best juice yield. That means taking your delicate greens like mint and wrapping them in your larger leaves like chard.
8. Always put the smaller ingredients in first, then add the larger items like celery and cucumbers so the larger bits can act like a chaser and push through all the smaller ingredients.
9. Unless specified, each of the following recipes will make approximately one 16-ounce serving.

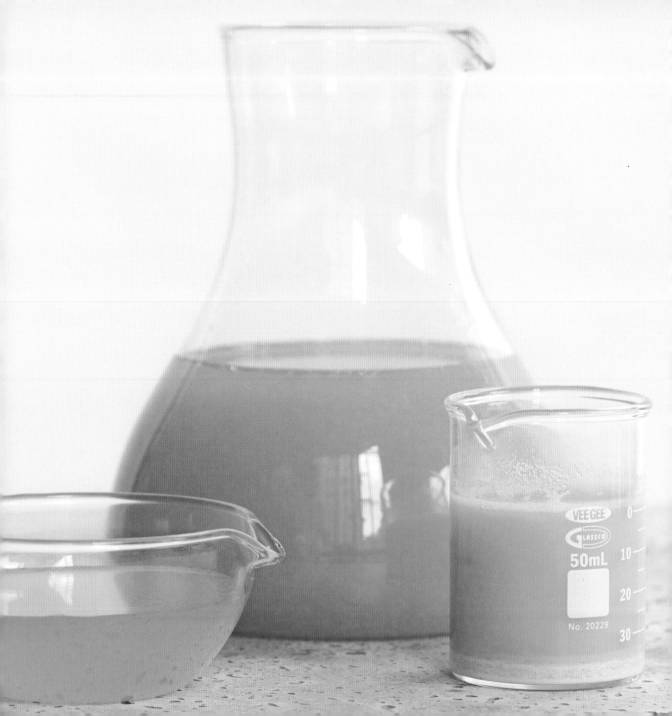

DETOX JUICES

These recipes are great ways to start your morning. They'll bring a level of alkaline into your body that wakes up the blood and gets you going. They are also great for getting your metabolism started and curbing your appetite. Having them a half hour before a meal is also a tasty way to get your digestion started right!

GRAPEFRUIT DETOX

7 oz. grapefruit juice

7 oz. water

2 oz. apple cider vinegar

1 pinch of cayenne pepper
(Optional)

Apple cider vinegar is one of my favorite ingredients. I cannot express how amazing it is. It helps to stimulate cardiovascular circulation and detoxification of the liver. It has been known to aid in weight loss, eliminating acne, and even reducing allergies and fighting yeast infections. Oh, and did I mention it seriously helps daytime fatigue? It's a natural energy booster—without the caffeine crash.

LEMON LIME DETOX

2 oz. lime juice

2 oz. lemon juice

6 oz. water

2 oz. apple cider vinegar

1 pinch cayenne pepper
   (Optional)

You will notice for this recipe I wrote out actual ounces of each ingredient. So, you should juice the citrus fruits and then add the other ingredients.

SPICY FRUIT

1 grapefruit (no skin)

2 cucumbers

1 thumb of ginger

Grapefruit is high in pectin, which has been known to help in the prevention of prostate and colon cancer.

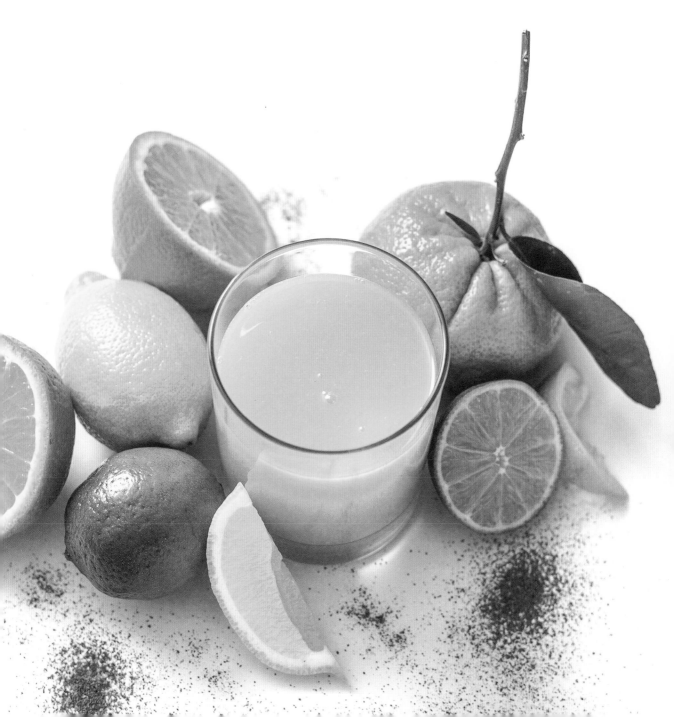

MASTER CLEANSE

2 tablespoons coconut palm
    sugar
4 tablespoons lemon
1 pinch cayenne
12 oz. of filtered water

This recipe is a take on the Master Cleanse.
While I disagree with their recommendation
of drinking this (and only this) for ten days, I
think this is a great way to start your day.

MASTER CLEANSE TEA

4 thin slices of ginger
½ lemon sliced, including peel
1 pinch cayenne

Place ingredients into a mug with 8 ounces
of hot water and enjoy. This is a great tea
for starting or ending your day. It helps with
digestion.

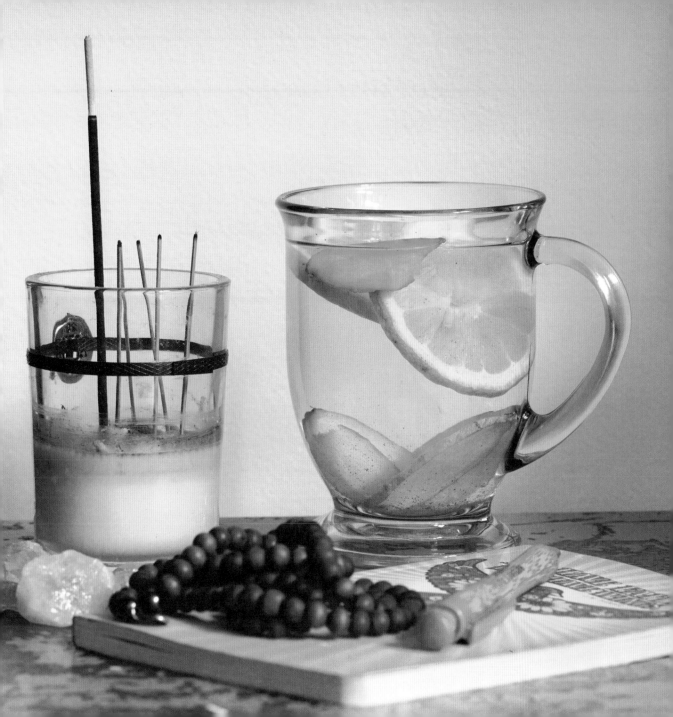

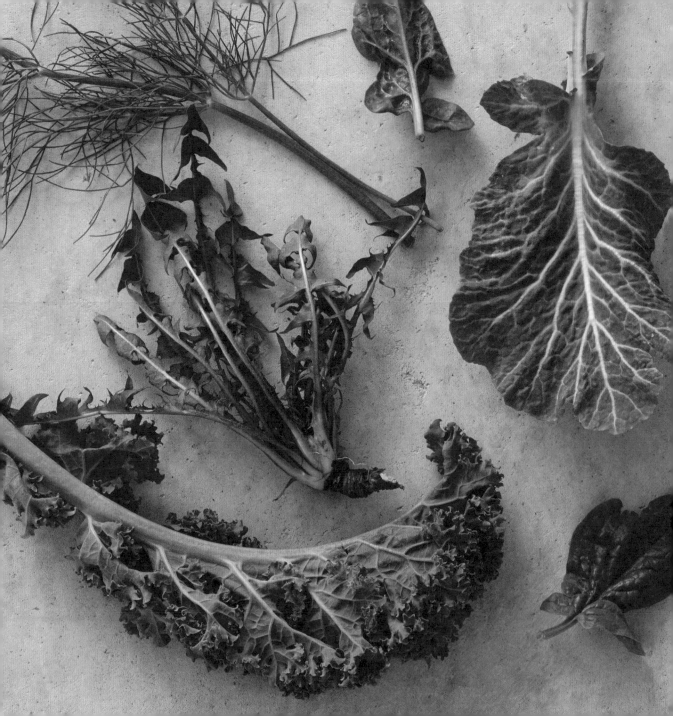

GREEN JUICES WITHOUT FRUIT

All these recipes are completely alkaline. There's no sugar in them, making these recipes a great place to start your morning. These are also good options if you're battling candida. Again, for any of the smaller, more delicate greens, you'll get more of a juice yield if you wrap them in the bigger greens before putting them through the juicer. It's also good to juice the leafier greens first and then follow that with a larger vegetable, like cucumber, so it pushes the greens through and you get a better yield.

CLEAN GREEN

5 collard leaves

5 chard leaves

3 stalks celery

½ cucumber

Collards are high in calcium, which is great for the bones and teeth! Some people shy away from green juice. They get scared it is going to taste too "green." I challenge you to play with these recipes. A correctly balanced all-green juice can taste light and refreshing. It is the most alkalizing thing you can do for you.

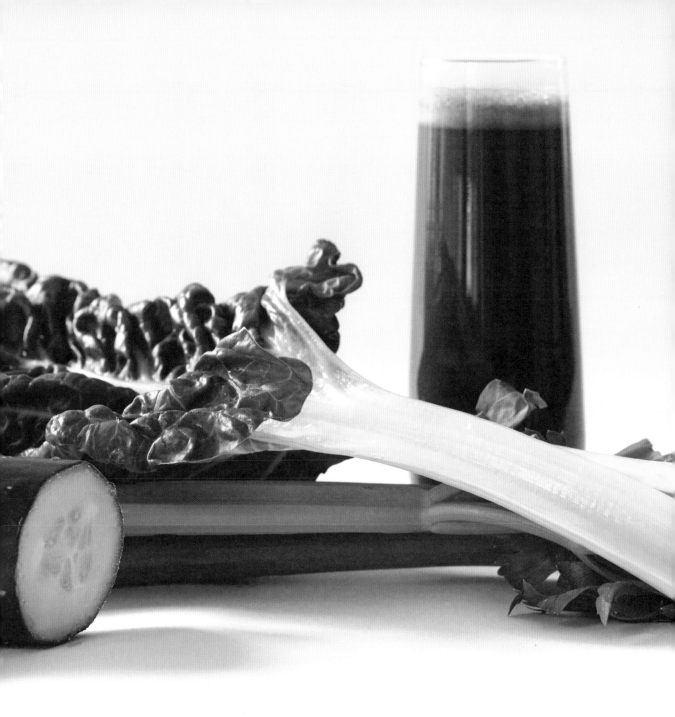

GREEN MONSTER

4 collard leaves

5 romaine leaves

1 cucumber

2 bunches parsley

1 lemon (no skin but leave white pith)

This is a great basic green juice. If you want to give it a kick, you can add a thumb of ginger or a pinch of cayenne pepper.

POPEYE

5 handfuls spinach

5 stalks celery

3 handfuls cilantro

Spinach is high in vitamin K, which is helpful for blood clotting. This is good for healing quicker and preventing excessive bleeding.

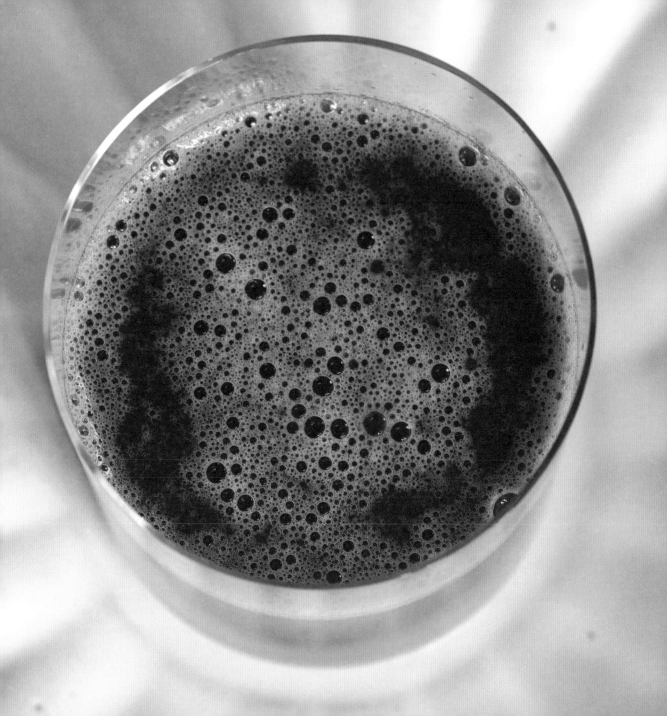

GREEN BUNNY

3 large chard leaves

2 handfuls spinach

4 large carrots

8 romaine leaves

1 stalk celery

This juice has a bit of sweetness to it from the carrot. It might be a nice place to start if you are looking to avoid the fruit or are nervous to jump right into an all-green juice.

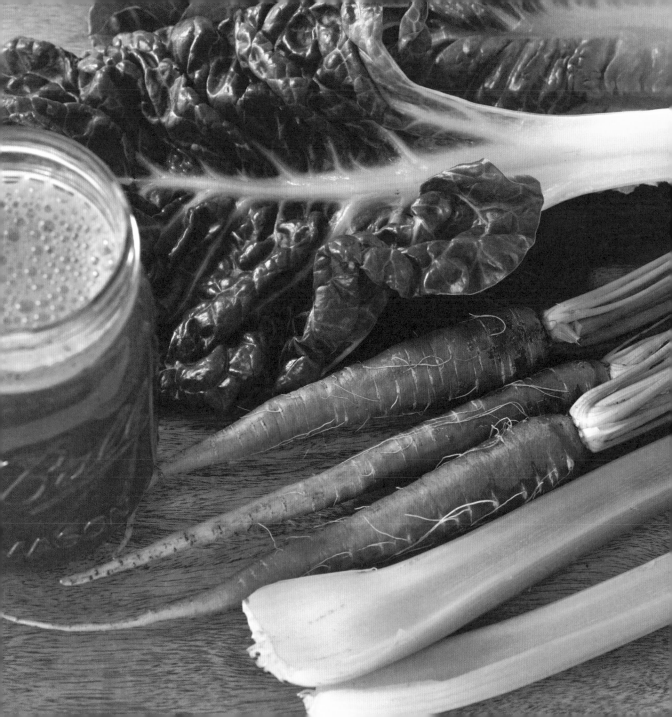

GROUNDING GREEN

1 bulb fennel

2 handfuls cilantro

2 large pieces burdock

3 large chard leaves

Burdock and fennel are two of my favorite ingredients. Not only do they taste great, but they are also both known for their healing properties. Burdock and fennel both act as diuretics and remove toxins from the body.

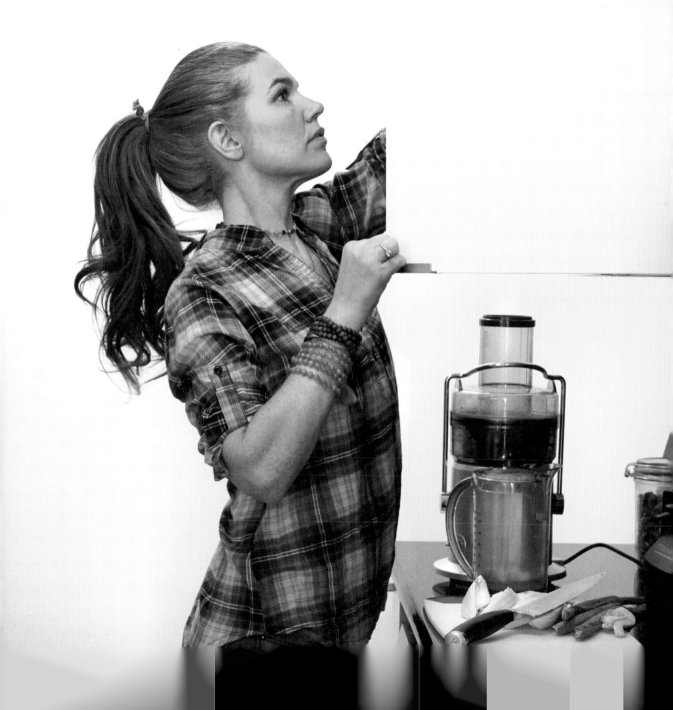

GINGER BLAST

1 full head romaine

1 whole cucumber

2 thumbs ginger

1 whole lime

2 kale leaves (with stems)

2 stalks celery

Ginger is one of my favorite vegetables. It adds a delicious spice to everything, but it is also incredibly healing. It reduces inflammation, stimulates circulation, and can help with digestion. I included 2 thumbs of ginger in this recipe, but if that is too strong for you, change it to 1 thumb.

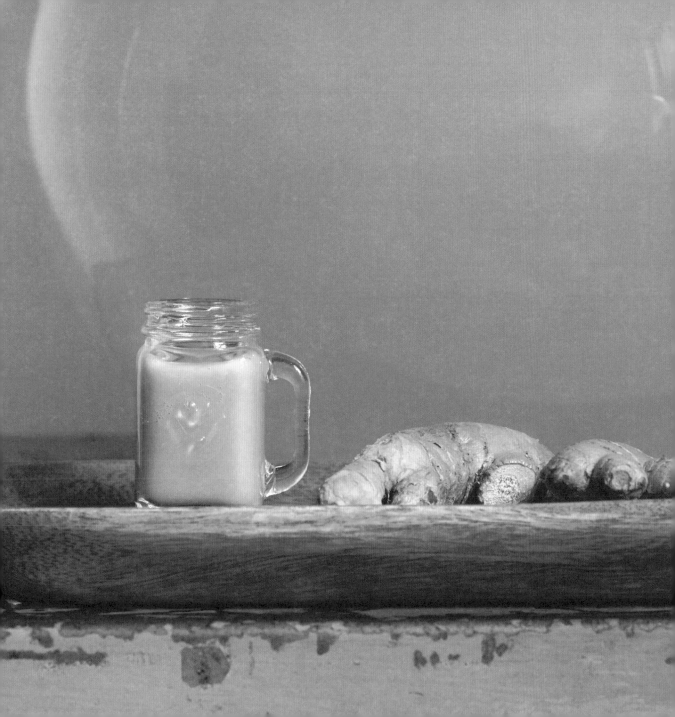

CLEAN BLOOD

1 handful cilantro

2 large chard leaves

1 cucumber

1 handful mint

Cilantro has long been said to be a huge helper in detoxification. Studies have shown that it helps to draw out the heavy metal toxins that people accumulate in their blood.

LEMON BURST

2 handfuls cilantro

8 kale leaves

1 large head romaine

1 lemon

Leaving the skin on when juicing lemons and limes is highly beneficial, as many nutrients are found in the skin. It does make the drink a little bitter, so if it is too much, only use half of the peel.

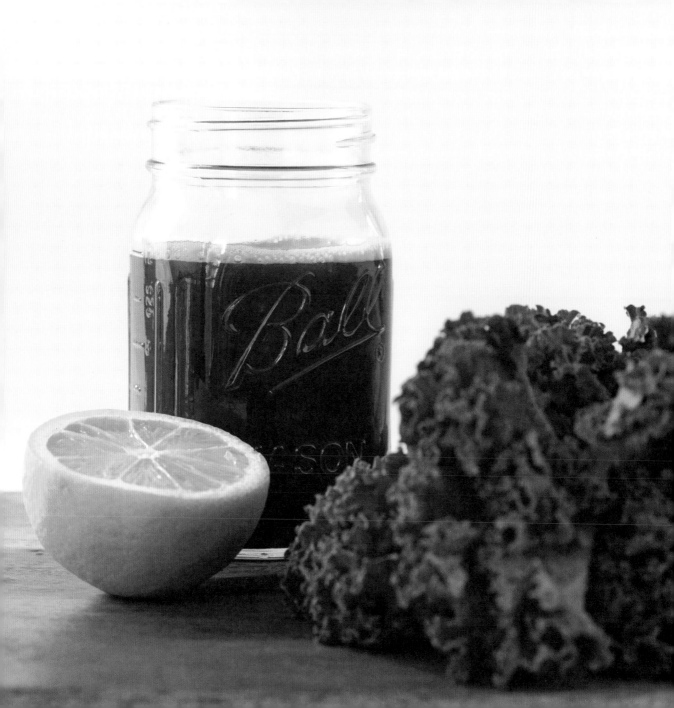

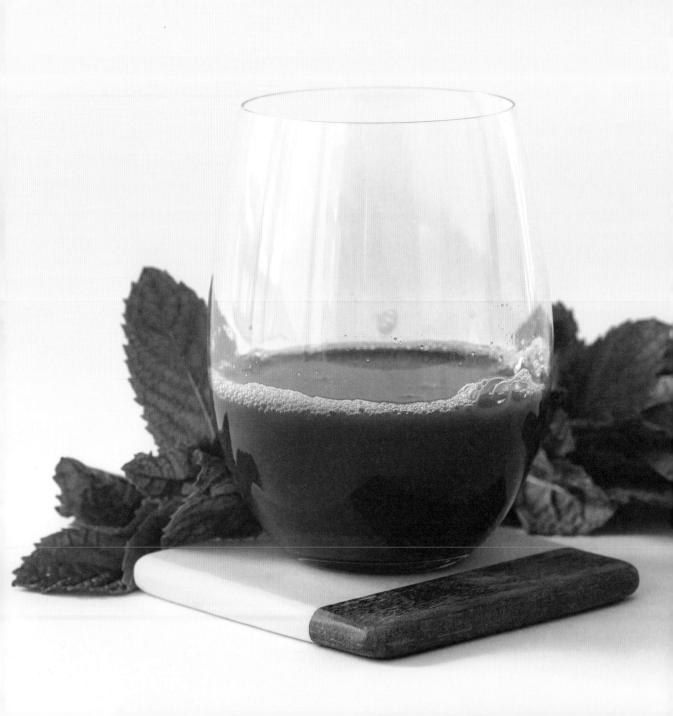

> Mint is known to help with digestion by relaxing the muscles and speeding up the process.

MINT DREAM

- 2 handfuls mint
- 3 large cucumbers
- 1 whole lime (leave ½ skin on)

This is a great summer drink. Highly refreshing and hydrating. Remember to put the mint in first then put the larger vegetables in after to help push the mint through.

MINTILICIOUS

- 2 handfuls mint
- 4 handfuls spinach
- 1 lime
- 10 romaine leaves
- 1 bulb fennel

Mint is great for digestion. It is known to soothe the stomach and it's a great way to wake you up!

SWEET SURPRISE

- 1 handful mint
- 3 chard leaves
- 1 bulb fennel

Fennel is quite sweet and adds a great candy-like flavor to juices. It taste a bit like licorice.

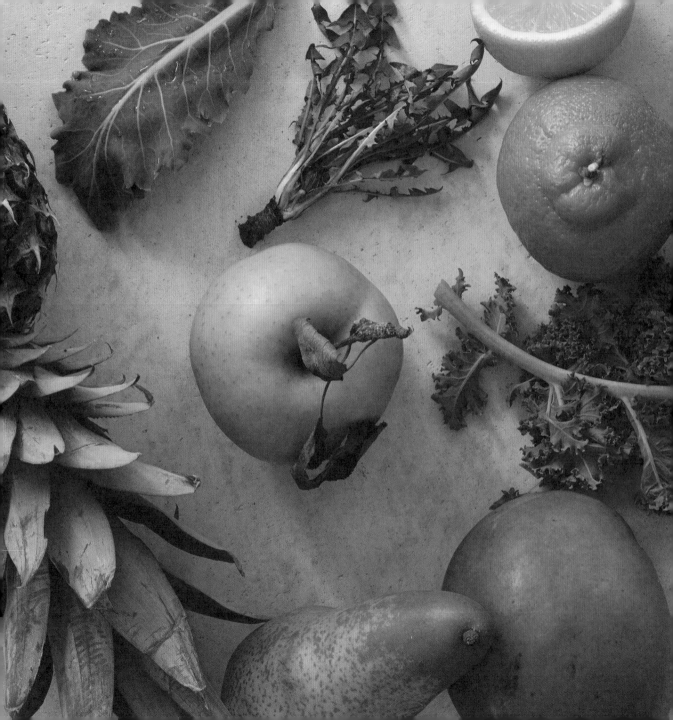

GREEN JUICES WITH FRUIT

With these juices, you'll get a little bit of sweetness. I chose to go light with the fruits, but if you want it sweeter then you can just add more fruit. Just be mindful of how much fruit you put in. To consider it a green juice, it should be at least a 3 to 1 ratio of greens to fruits. The more bitter the green you choose, the more likely you'll need to add in more fruit. These are great for children and people who are new to juicing.

GREEN BASIL

4 kale leaves

2 handfuls basil

3 handfuls spinach

1 handful dandelion

1 cucumber

½ green apple

Basil is quite possibly the tastiest herb on Earth. I love it with both sweet drinks and savory drinks. It's easy to understand why it's known as the king of herbs! Not only is it delicious, but it has anti-inflammatory and antibacterial properties.

SWEET & SPICY

1 head romaine

3 chard leaves

½ green apple

1 handful parsley

1 whole lemon

1 thumb ginger

This is a great spicy drink, but if you are looking for something a bit more mild, add less ginger.

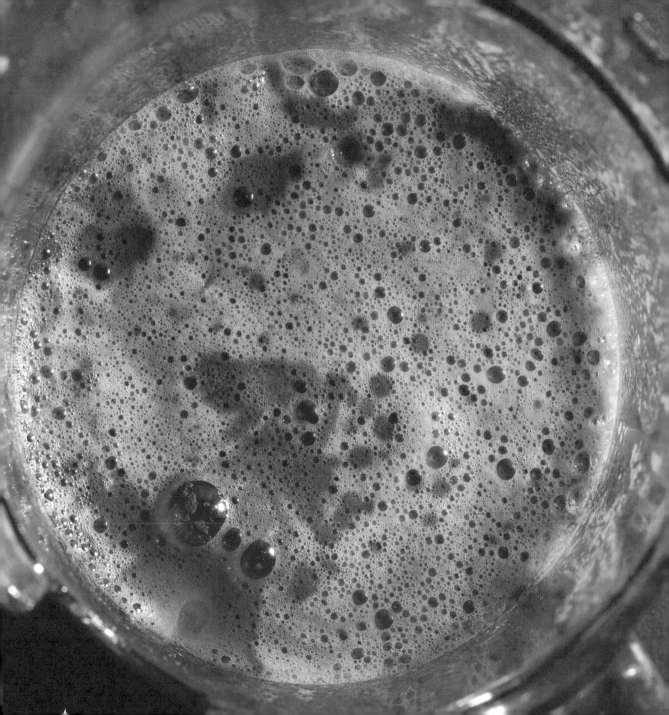

GREEN WARRIOR

¼ green apple

3 stalks celery

1 handful spinach

2 kale leaves

1 handful mint

½ head romaine

½ cucumber

Green apples are a great way to sweeten your juice without spiking your sugar levels. They are a little tart, which also adds a nice layer to your juice!

GREEN CANDY

1 stalk celery

½ pear

1 bulb fennel

1 handful mint

5 chard leaves

This is a terrific green juice for kids. Sweetness is derived not only from the pear, but the fennel as well.

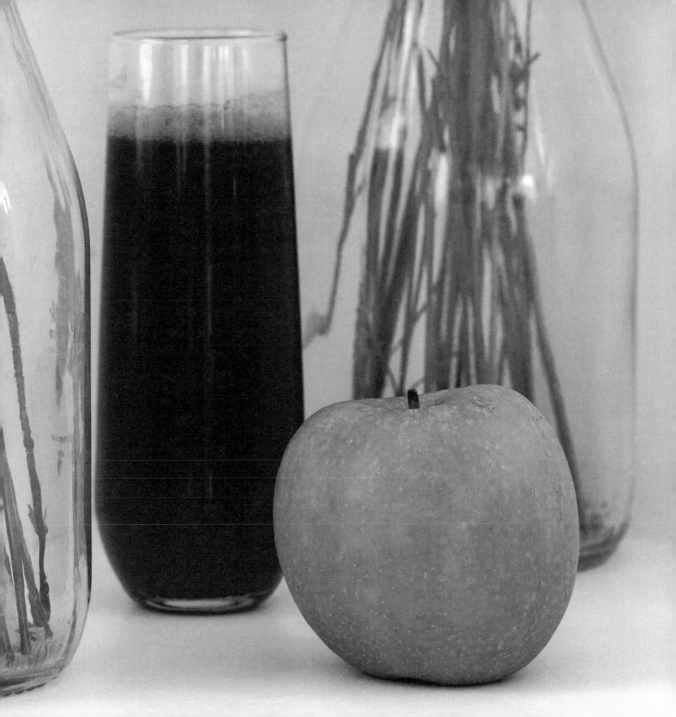

GREEN BURST

2 stalks celery

2 pears

1 bulb fennel

1 handful parsley

2 kale leaves

½ lemon (skin on)

Parsley is a natural blood balancer; this protects against insulin resistance. It is also high in antioxidant vitamins, including A, C, and E.

DETOX ME

10 chard leaves

4 handfuls cilantro

1 pear

Cilantro is great for heavy metal detoxification. Heavy metal toxification is one of the many issues we get from eating nonorganic foods.

Recipe Notes

DANDY JUICE

½ head romaine

½ bunch dandelion

1 large cucumber

¼ pear

1 orange

Dandelion is great for helping with digestion. It can be helpful with elimination. If you have a problem going to the bathroom, dandelion can help.

AMAZING GREENS

4 stalks celery

2 handfuls cilantro

3 large chard leaves

3 kale leaves

½ lime

1 small handful of dandelion

½ pear

Dandelion is a natural diuretic; it helps eliminate toxic substances in the kidneys. It is quite bitter, though, so you want to be careful of using too much.

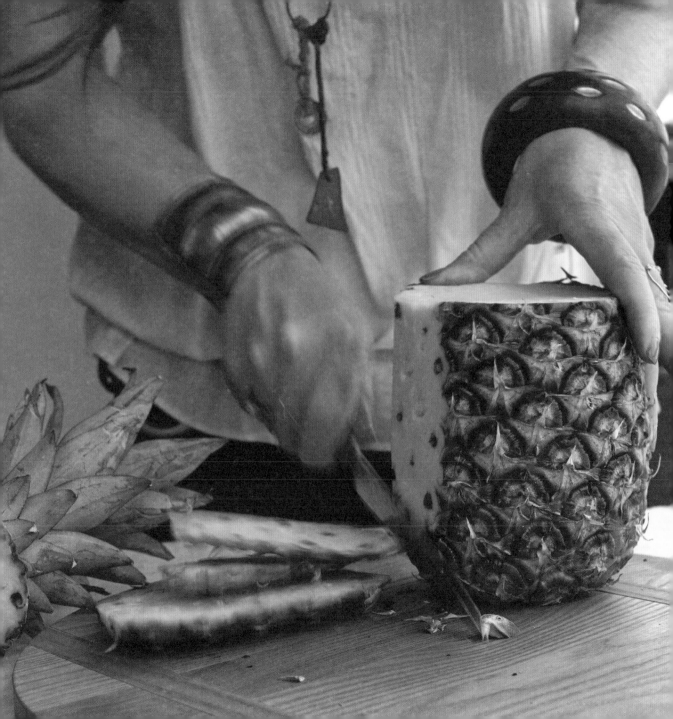

TROPICAL GREEN

1 head romaine

6 kale leaves

3 handfuls pineapple, cubed

2 handfuls basil

Pineapple is high in bromelain, which is a beneficial digestive aid. It is also anti-inflammatory and contains enzymes that help to digest fat and turn it to waste.

MANGO MADNESS

1 head romaine

3 kale leaves

2 handfuls pineapple, cubed

2 handfuls cilantro

1 mango

Mango is not only delicious, but it is also high in iron. This is particularly useful for people who are anemic.

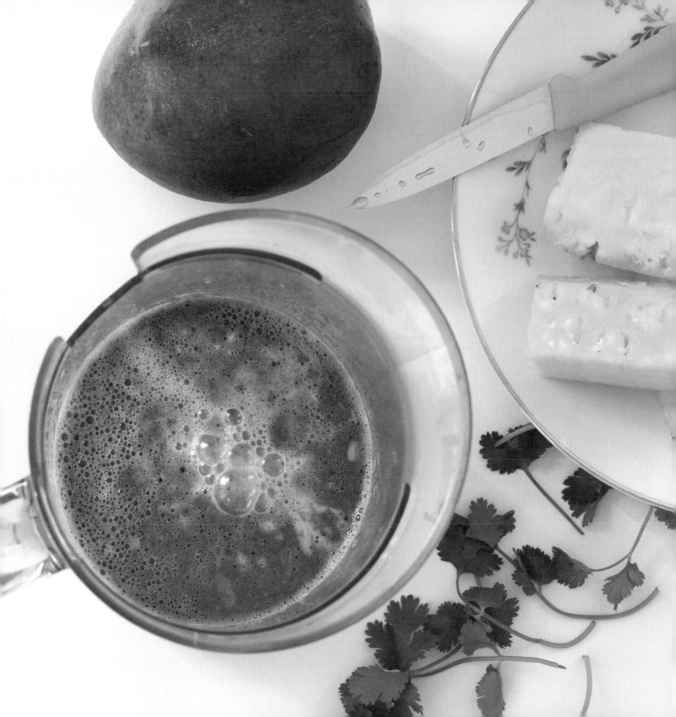

TROPICAL MINT

2 cucumbers

4 kale leaves

2 handfuls pineapple, cubed

2 handfuls mint

Kale is known as the king of healthy greens. It is loaded with vitamins A, K, C, and B6, and is packed with minerals, calcium, magnesium, and potassium. This is a great recipe to sneak in all those nutritional benefits, while feeling like you are having a treat.

GREEN MELON

2 heads romaine

½ cantaloupe (with seeds)

3 handfuls pineapple, cubed

3 handfuls mint

This is great for a hot summer day. It will be a very hydrating and refreshing drink.

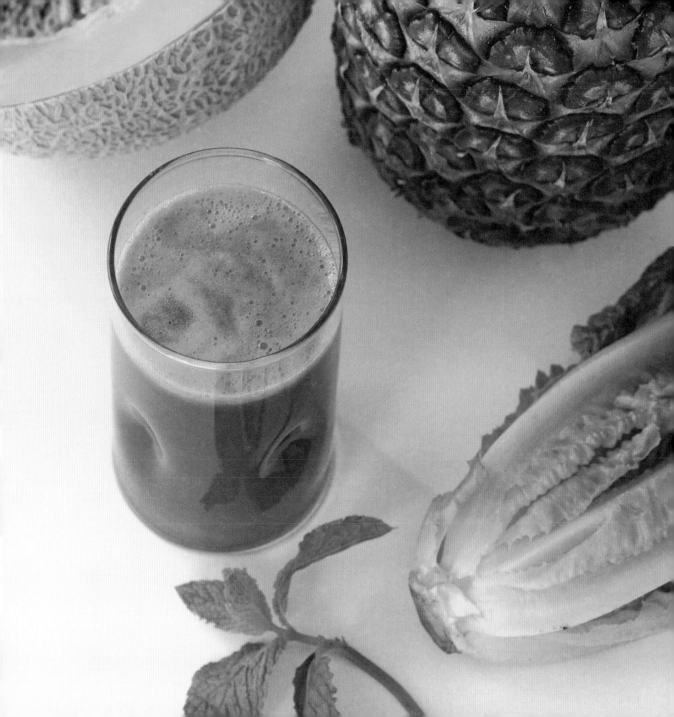

MAGICAL LOVE

¼ cantaloupe

2 kiwi

1 cucumber

Loaded with vitamin A, your skin will be thanking you for this delicious treat!

STARBURST

2 kiwi

½ cantaloupe

You will swear you are eating candy. You can also freeze it and make it into Popsicles. The kids will be begging you for more!

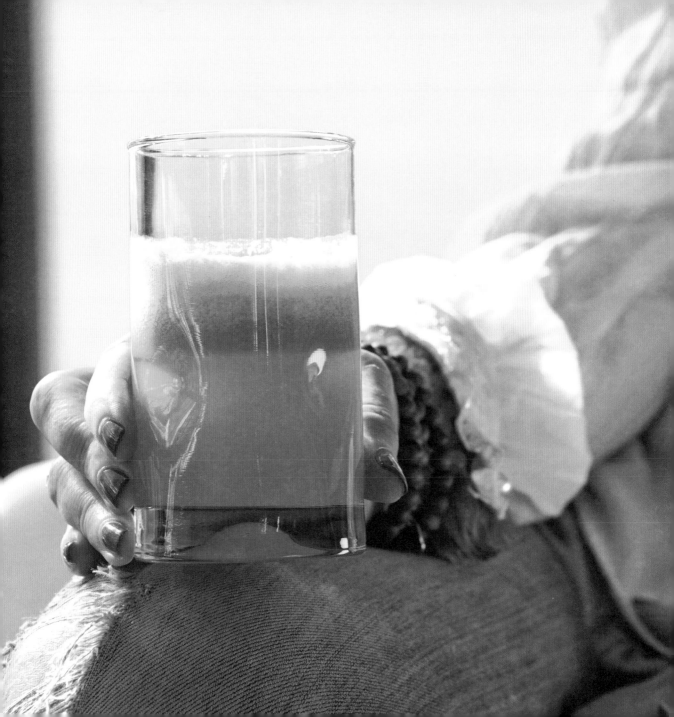

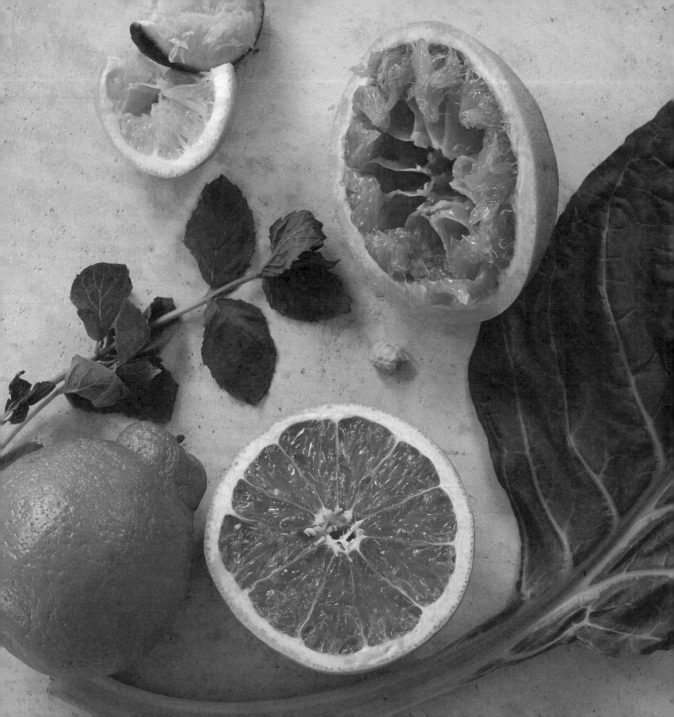

GREEN JUICES WITH CITRUS

These recipes are great for those new to juicing. When it comes to lemon and lime, when you're juicing you can leave the skin on since there's more nutrition in the skin than there is in the fruit. But if you find the juice is too bitter with the entire rind on, then feel free to take half the skin off, but remove all the skin when it comes to tangerines, oranges, and grapefruits. Do leave as much of the pith (the white rind) as you can. For kiwis, the skin should be left on.

GREEN ORANGE

1 orange

5 kale leaves

½ bulb fennel

2 handfuls spinach

1 cucumber

As we all know, oranges are a great source of vitamin C. A medium-sized orange contains more than 70 percent of your daily requirements of vitamin C.

ORANGE CRUSH

2 oranges

6 kale leaves

8 stalks basil

6 chard leaves

1 cucumber

Often people mistake oranges for an acidic fruit, but they are actually filled with alkaline minerals that help balance the body when digested. Similar to lemons, once digested, they're a highly alkaline fruit!

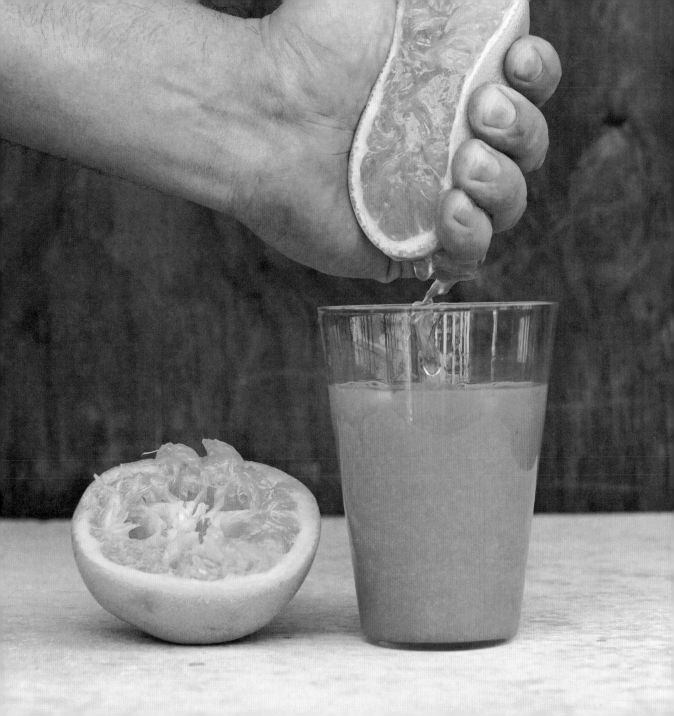

VIBRANT LIME

5 kale leaves

2 handfuls cilantro

½ grapefruit

½ lime

Remember to take 1 handful of cilantro and wrap it in 2 kale leaves. Repeat with the second bunch and the remaining 2 kale leaves.

BLISSFULLY BASIL

2 large handfuls basil

2 cucumbers

1 orange

Put the basil in first and then place the cucumbers in the blender or juicer so you get the most juice possible.

KIWI LOVE

2 kiwis (skin on)

3 stalks celery

4 chard leaves

1 tangerine (no skin, but leave pith)

Although kiwis can taste quite sweet, they are actually low on the glycemic index and have high amounts of fiber. This means they will not spike your sugar levels and won't be stored as fat!

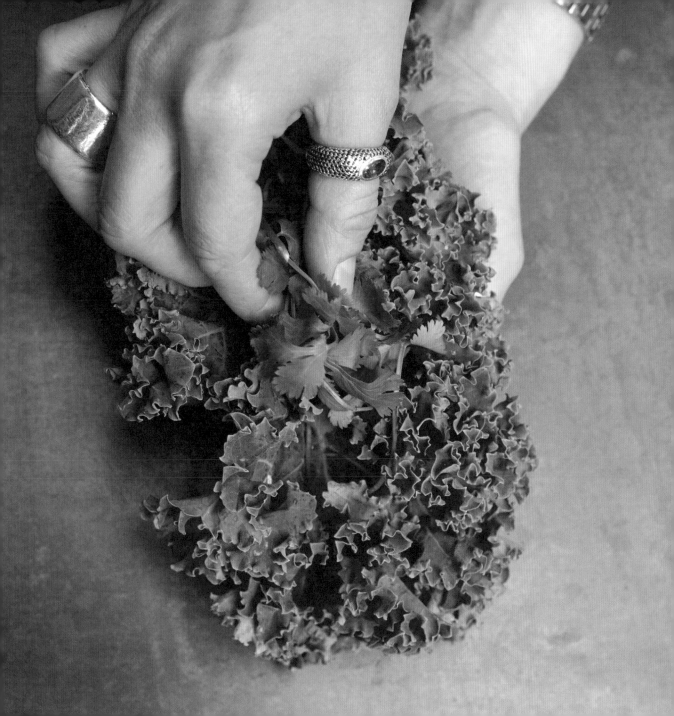

DELICATE GREENS

4 kale leaves

6 chard leaves

1 handful cilantro

1 handful mint

1 handful dandelion

½ lemon

1 orange

This recipe has a large amount of smaller herbs. When you juice the bigger leaves, like kale and chard, wrap them around the smaller herbs. This will help you get more juice from the smaller herbs. Leave the skin on the lemon and end with the orange, no skin.

GREEN LICORICE

10 chard leaves

4 handfuls cilantro

1 pear

½ bulb fennel

½ grapefruit

Chard is a powerhouse of nutrition. It is loaded with vitamins K, C, A, and E.

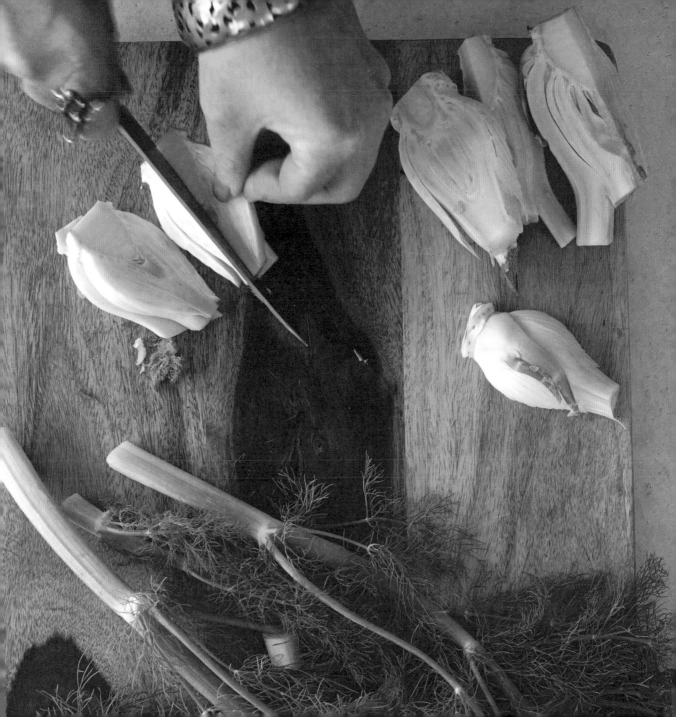

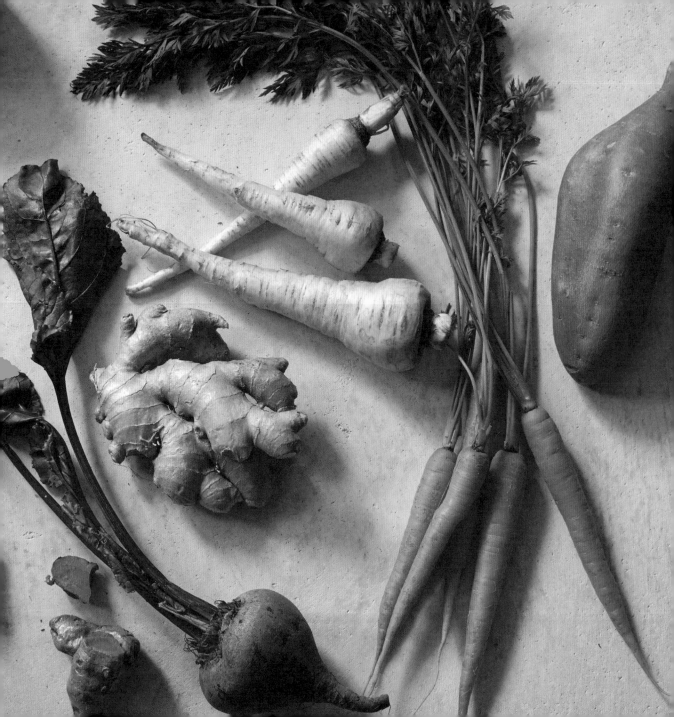

ROOT JUICES

These recipes are based in root vegetables. They're very satisfying and though many don't have fruit, you will be surprised at how sweet and delicious they are. They make great dessert juices!

ORANGE PEAR

12 inches burdock

½ pear

2 large carrots

Burdock is high in vitamin B6, which is good for keeping your brain working and your moods balanced. Burdock root is also high in potassium, which is important for heart function and muscle contraction. Potassium also counterbalances the overconsumption of salt.

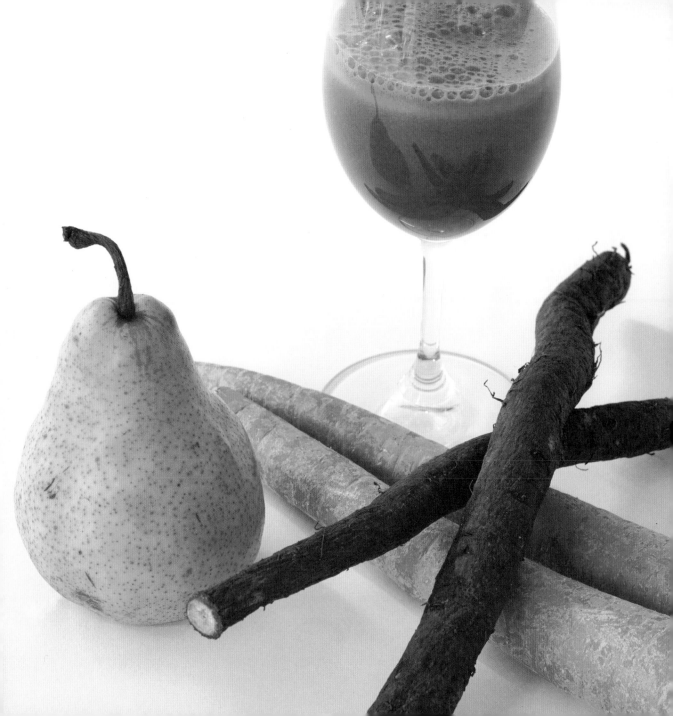

BEETS ME

3 beets

3 carrots

4 stalks celery

1 thumb ginger

Beets are seriously one of nature's great aphrodisiacs! Their high levels of boron help with the production of sex hormones.

SWEETIE PIE

1 sweet potato

6 handfuls spinach

2 large carrots

1 dash cinnamon

This will literally taste like Thanksgiving in a glass. A wonderful treat, filled with vitamins A, C, E, and B6.

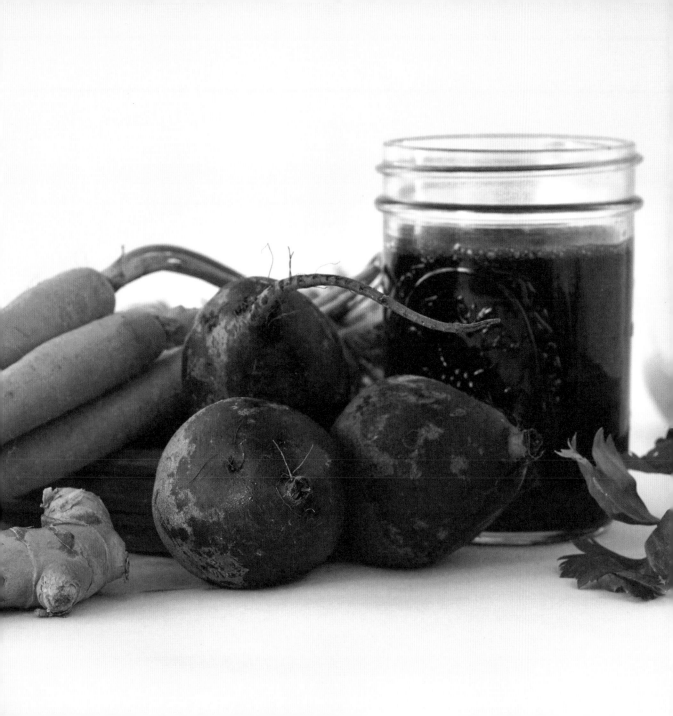

LIQUID CANDY

2 parsnips
2 zucchinis
12 inches burdock
3 kale leaves

Parsnips are an incredible vegetable to add to juice. They are sweet and packed with folate. Folate intake is especially important for pregnant women.

ORANGE JULIUS

4 parsnips
1 orange

This is truly heaven in a cup! Parsnips are able to fill you up without the release of ghrelin, which is a "hunger" hormone. This can really help with keeping you satiated, while also tasting delicious. This is a great one when you are looking for a treat that is also good for you. I will often have this one for dessert!

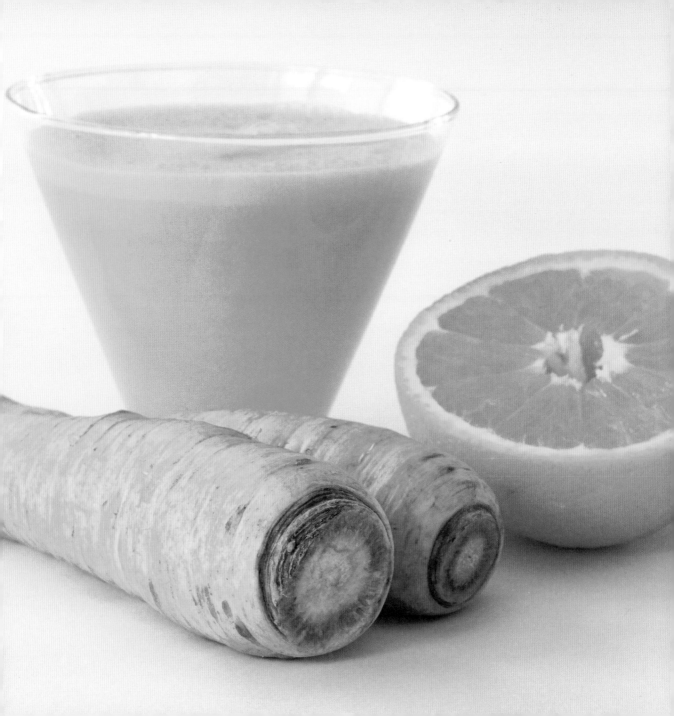

SWEET GINGER

2 parsnips

1 orange

¼ sweet potato

2 thumbs ginger

1 head romaine

A great juice for someone looking for something spicy and sweet. Parsnips are high in vitamin C, folate, and manganese. If it is too spicy, use half the amount of ginger.

GREEN SURPRISE

1 cucumber

6 inches burdock

½ zucchini

½ fennel bulb

1 large handful mint

¼ pear

Zucchini juice is often associated with anti-aging. It is rich in flavonoid polyphenolic antioxidants, which reduce harmful oxygen-derived free radicals from the body that are known to cause aging. It also cleanses the kidneys and blood vessels.

BURDOCK · CARROTS · BERRIES
BEETS · PARSNIPS · BANANAS · AVOCADOS · LIME
CELERY · PINEAPPLES · PEARS · KALE

ORANGE

MANGO · TOMATOES · APPLES
GREENS · KIWI · BASIL · SWISS CHARD · PARSLEY
CUCUMBERS · GINGER · LEMON · MINT
FENNEL · ROMAINE · DANDELION

SWEET ROOTS

1 thumb turmeric
12 inches burdock
12 inches parsnip
2 large carrots
1½ heads romaine

Turmeric is known for its anti-inflammatory benefits. Because of this, it is thought to help in the fight against cancer, arthritis, Alzheimer's, and many other diseases.

SPICY LOVE

3 zucchinis
1½ thumbs turmeric
1 thumb ginger
3 kale leaves
1 orange

Turmeric is a powerful player in the health world. It is highly anti-inflammatory and is often used for various ailments. It is spicy, so start with a little and then add more.

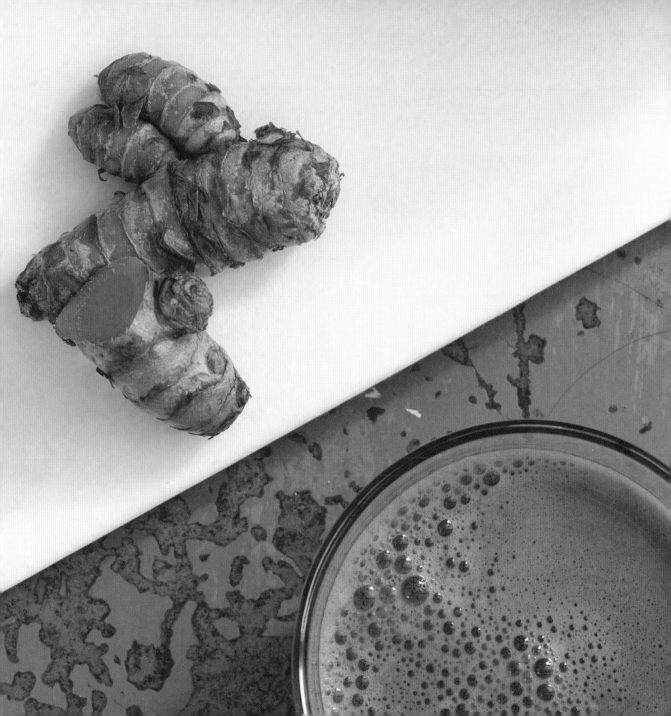

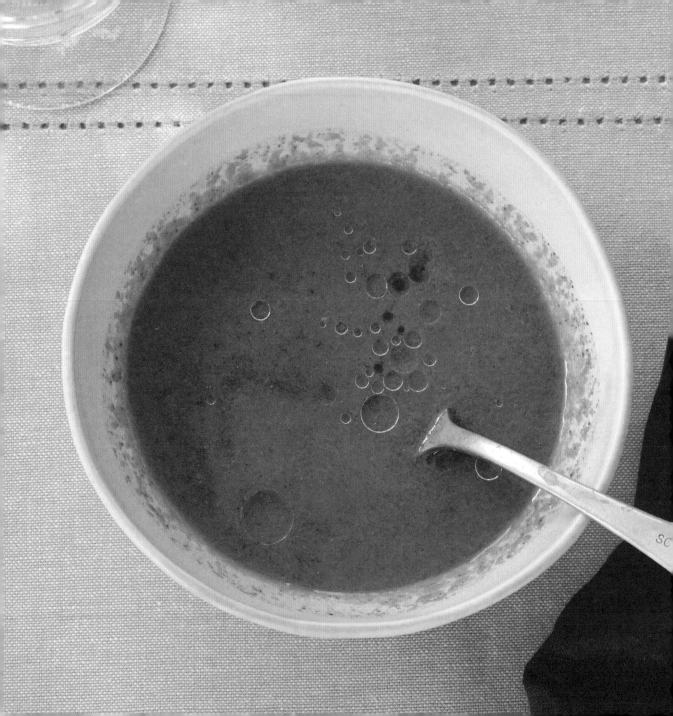

SAVORY JUICES (A.K.A. SOUPS)

These are savory juice options. Think of them like soups. You can drink these out of a bottle, but some might be nice to serve in a bowl. I highly recommend having at least one of these while on a cleanse to balance out the fruit and sugar in the sweeter juices. It's also a great way to satisfy your savory craving.

BASIL BOOGEY

2 tomatoes

2 stalks basil

1 zucchini

1 clove garlic

1 stalk celery

2 kale leaves

Wrap the basil inside of the kale to get the best yield. You can also stick the garlic inside the zucchini before you juice it. This will allow you to get more from the garlic.

G'SNAPS V8

¼ red bell pepper

8 stalks celery

1½ tomatoes

1 kale leaf

1 small handful dandelion

A zesty and vibrant juice that will enable you to get many of your veggies in for the day.

SPICY RED

2 small tomatoes

½ clove or 1 small clove garlic

1 zucchini

This is a great red soup base. You can get creative and add different spices and vegetables. If you are looking to make it spicy, add cayenne pepper. If you want something heavier, add olive oil or avocado. These are just a few examples. Get creative and play.

CLASSIC KALE

2 small tomatoes

1½ large or 3 small cloves garlic

1 zucchini

1 large handful cilantro

2 kale leaves

1 stalk celery

Go light with the garlic. I suggest a lot in this recipe. Start with less, and see if you want to add. Wrap the garlic in your kale or inside your zucchini. Save the celery for last so it can push the remaining ingredients through.

RACE IT RED

1 zucchini

1 tomato

6 basil leaves

1 clove garlic

1 kale leaf

1 pinch salt

1 teaspoon oil (optional)

½ cup water

4 sprigs oregano

This is a delicious soup that can be made heavier by adding in a bit of cold-pressed, organic virgin olive oil. If you are looking to avoid the fat, skip the oil.

Recipe Notes

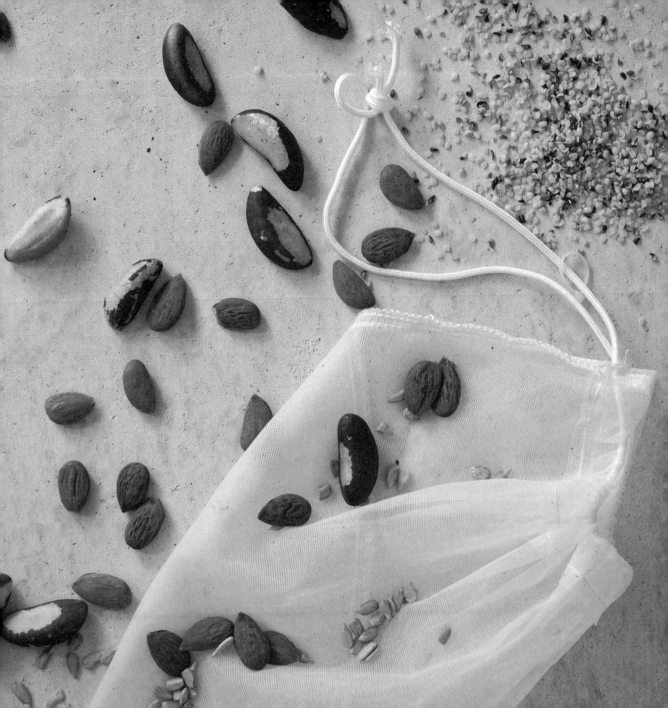

MILKS

All the milks in this section can be used for bases for smoothies or for your cereal. They are easy to make, especially the seed milks. They also add protein and fiber and make the smoothies extra creamy and delicious!

NUT MILKS

It is important to wash your nuts after they have been soaking. After that, place them in the blender with the proper amount of water. Start your blender on low and slowly move up to high. Blend them for about a minute or two. You want to make sure the nuts are all blended down, but don't let it sit too long or your blender could heat the milk. After that, take your nut milk bag and place it above a large bowl. You will slowly pour your blender contents into the nut milk bag. The milk will start pouring into the bowl. Gently squeeze the bag to get out all of the liquid. Pour this mixture back into your blender. Then add in the other ingredients. Blend for about one minute. Feel free to store the extra liquid in a mason jar. It will keep for three to four days. If you have a dehydrator, take the nut pulp and put it in a tray to make into flour. After it is dry, put it in the blender to break it down into flour. If you don't have a dehydrator, you can use an oven on the lowest temperature with the door slightly open.

SEED MILKS

All of the above information remains the same, but what is great about seed milk is you do not have to strain it. Follow the above instructions until you get to the nut milk bag. This can save a lot of time and hassle.

Tips & Tricks for Milks

Before Making Milks—*Please read this before making any of the milk recipes. It will help you get the most out of all your nuts!*

1. If you are strapped for time, go with seed milks. You do not have to strain them so it takes a step out.
2. Soaking times:
   a. Almonds—about 8 hours
   b. Brazil nuts—about 4 hours
   c. Hemp seeds—don't soak
   d. Coconut—don't soak
   e. Sunflower seeds—8 hours
3. Please note that soaking nuts and seeds is very important. They contain enzymes that prohibit you from getting all the nutrition they offer, but by soaking them you release the nutrients, making them better available to digest.
4. Notes on soaking: Put your nuts or seeds in filtered water with just enough to cover them and then cover the jar and place it in your fridge. Add a pinch of sea salt. Store for times mentioned above and then rinse. Wash them until the water runs clear.
5. Unless specified, each of the following recipes will make approximately one 16-20 ounce serving.
6. If you want the milk heavier, you can lessen the water and if you want it thinner, then add more.
7. Always use filtered water!

👈 Unflavored Plain Milks

All of the milk recipes are designed with the idea that you are using them alone, either for a milk or cream replacement. If you are using nut milks in a recipe for a smoothie, you should be using unflavored milks. You can easily convert any of the following recipes by leaving out all of the added ingredients and just using the nuts or seeds and water.

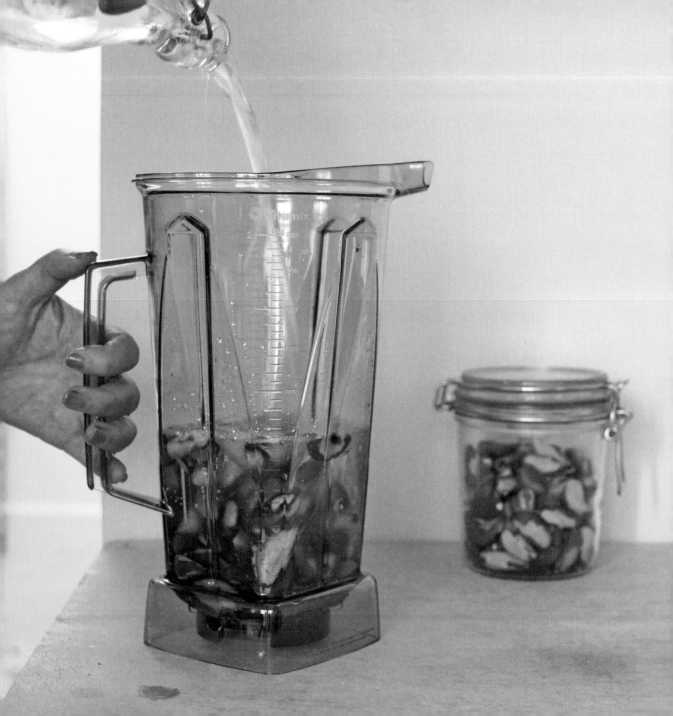

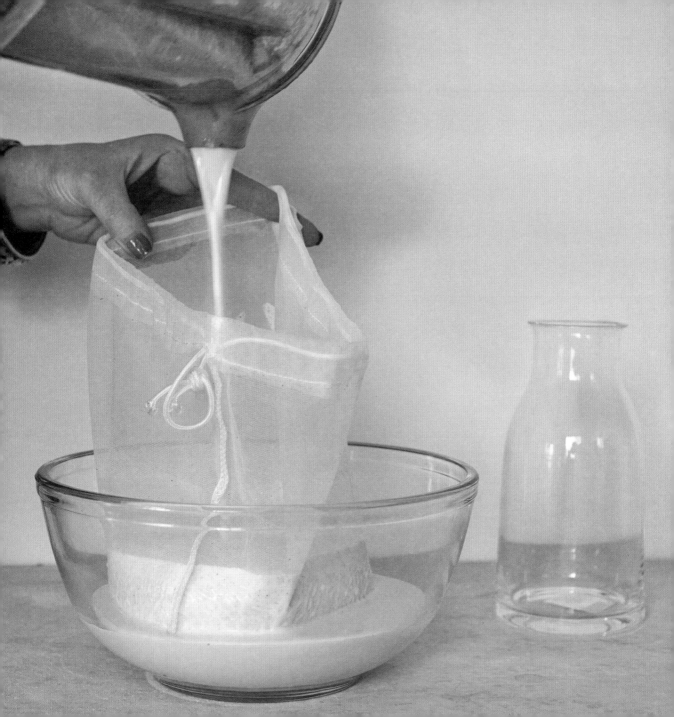

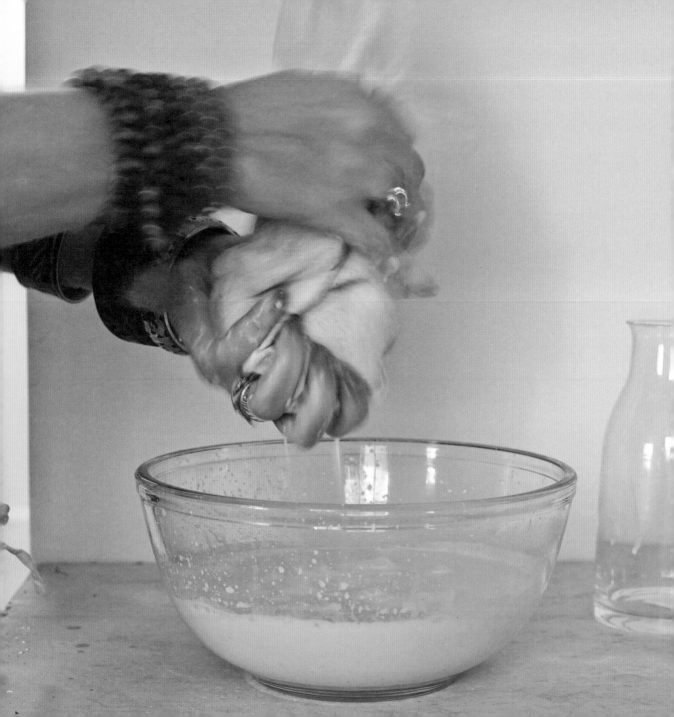

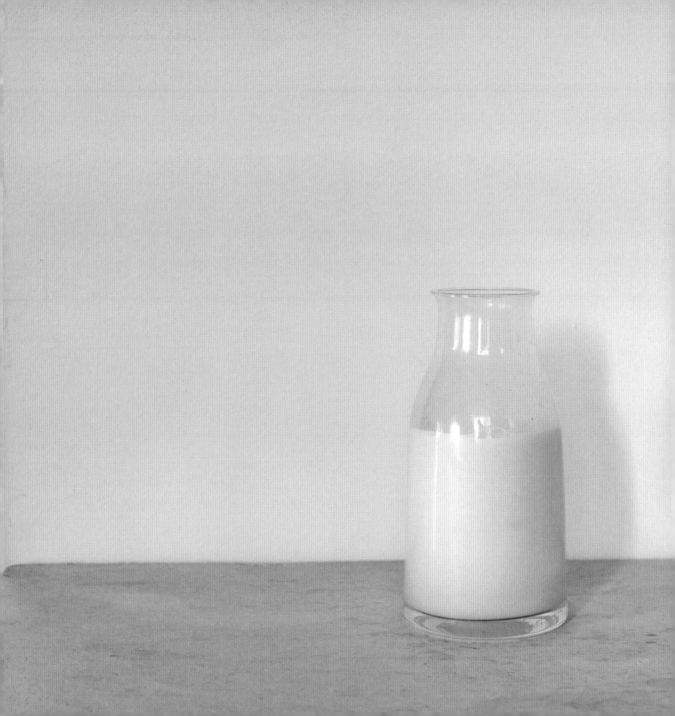

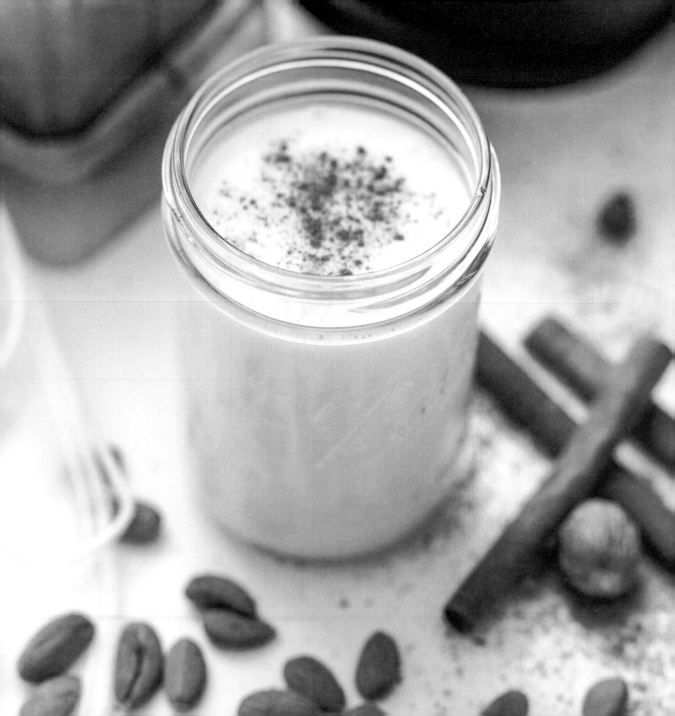

ALMOND MILK

1 cup raw almonds

3 cups filtered water

1 teaspoon vanilla extract

2 tablespoons coconut palm sugar

1 pinch sea salt

Almonds are high in fiber and protein. They are the least acidic nut. They are best when they are unpasteurized. Usually that means they are from California, Italy, or Spain.

BRAZIL NUT MILK

1 cup raw Brazil nut

3 cups filtered water

4 dates

1 pinch salt

Brazil nuts contain the highest levels of the trace mineral selenium. This is a very important antioxidant and it has been linked to reducing risks of cancer.

HEMP MILK

⅔ cup hemp seeds

2 cups water

4 dates

1 tablespoon cinnamon

1 pinch salt

Hemps seeds are a great form of digestible fiber. They also contain all nine of the essential amino acids. This is important because your body needs them to build muscle. Your body cannot do this on its own.

COCONUT MILK

⅔ cup coconut flakes

1 teaspoon coconut oil

2 cups filtered water

1 banana

Coconuts are said to reduce fat and add energy. It is also sweet without spiking your glycemic index.

SUNFLOWER MILK

½ cup sunflower

1½ cups filtered water

3 dates

1 thumb ginger

½ teaspoon vanilla

1 pinch salt

This is a great milk for children. Sunflower seeds are a good source of proteins and they have amino acids such as tryptophan that are essential for growth.

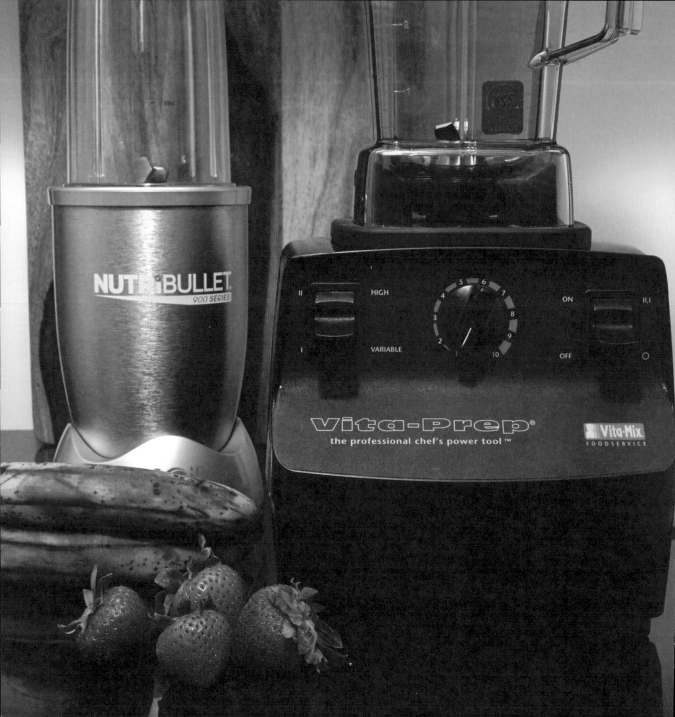

SOME TIPS FOR SMOOTHIES

Before Blending—*Please read this before making any of the smoothie recipes. It will help you get the most out of all your fruits and vegetables!*

1. Wash everything thoroughly.
2. Unlike juicing, remove all the skins for your citrus fruits. Leave as much of the pith on as possible.
3. Ginger—it's also great if you leave the skin on.
4. 1 handful = 1 packed cup.
5. It is great to use frozen fruits in these recipes. This is an easier way to always have them in stock, and the frozen quality creates a nice thick texture.
6. Start with your liquids and your softer fruits; this will make it easier on the blender.
7. Always make sure your blender is on low when starting and gradually move it to high.
8. If the blender gets stuck, slowly add a small bit of filtered water.
9. These are great places to add the superfoods, oils, and spices. Be creative!
10. Unless specified, each of the following recipes will make approximately one 16-ounce serving.

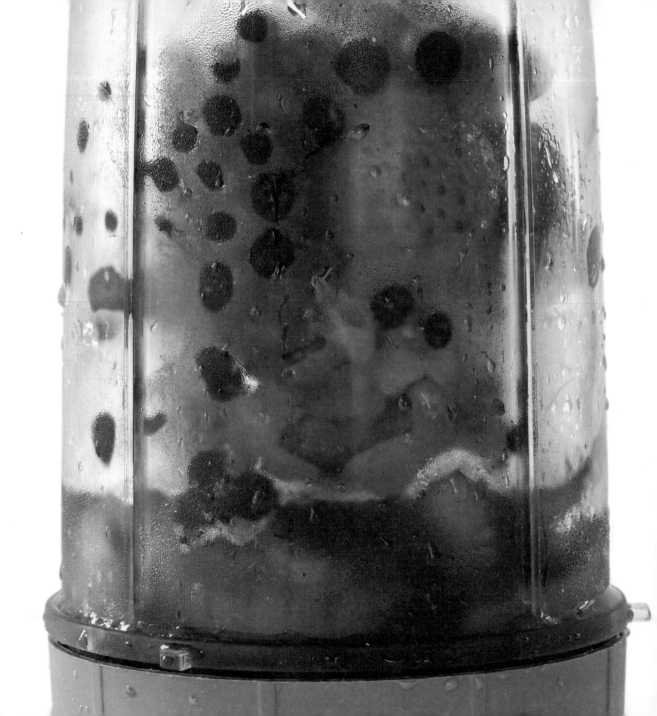

SMOOTHIES WITH FRUIT

These are great for kids. They're also delicious as desserts. It is often difficult to get kids to eat all their fruits and vegetables, but the following recipes makes it a cinch. They taste so good your children will be asking for more! If you're on a cleanse, I would recommend having only one to two maximum per day. For these recipes, it is nice for some of the fruits to be frozen. This gives a bit of a thicker texture, and freezing them also makes it easier to keep your kitchen stocked with fruit without worrying about waste!

KICK IT ORANGE

½ orange

¼ green apple

1 cup water

½ cup ice

6 sprigs cilantro

This is a very light and refreshing smoothie. Its texture will be more of a slushie than a typical smoothie.

MINTY APPLE

¼ fennel bulb

½ apple

5 sprigs mint

½ cup ice

1 cup filtered water

2 kale leaves

This is super refreshing without being too sweet. Fennel gives it a nice licorice taste and is great for zapping free radicals that lead to disease!

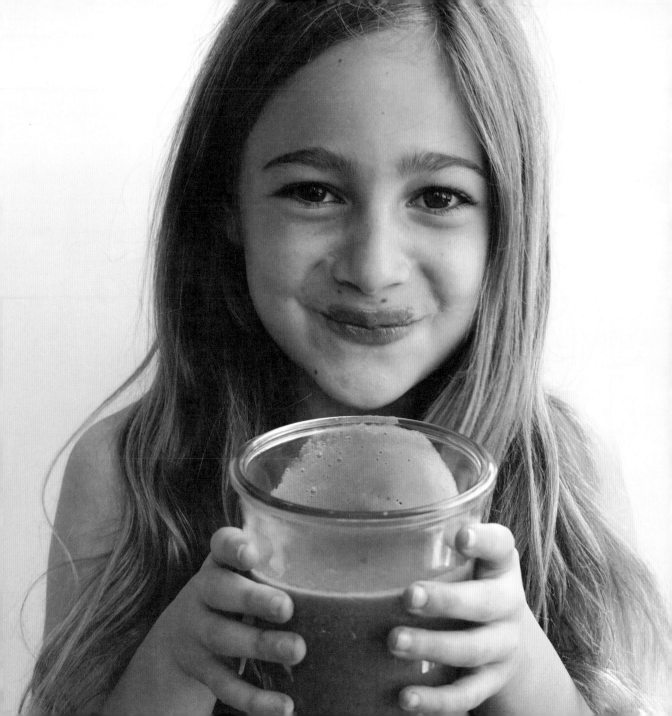

BASIL KISS

⅔ cup mango

⅓ cup strawberry

2 handfuls spinach

½ cucumber

5 basil leaves

½ cup filtered water

Yummy. The basil adds an extra interesting taste level to this dreamy concoction. If making this one for kids, you might want to leave out the basil.

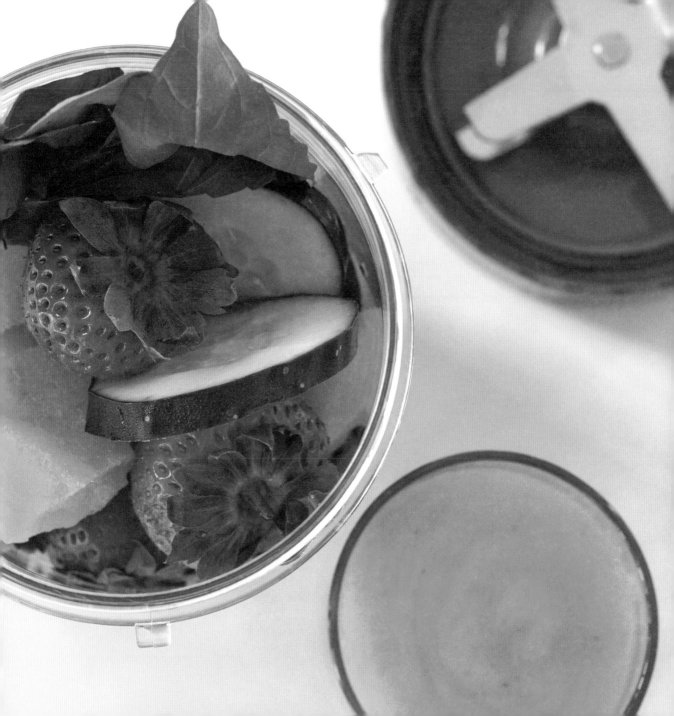

BRAZILIAN KICK

1 package unsweetened açai
1 pear
1 handful spinach
½ zucchini
½ cup mango
5 sprigs mint
½ cup water

It is said that açai contains more antioxidant capacity than all the other berries! When buying it, make sure you are getting the unsweetened version, as the others have unnecessary added sugars.

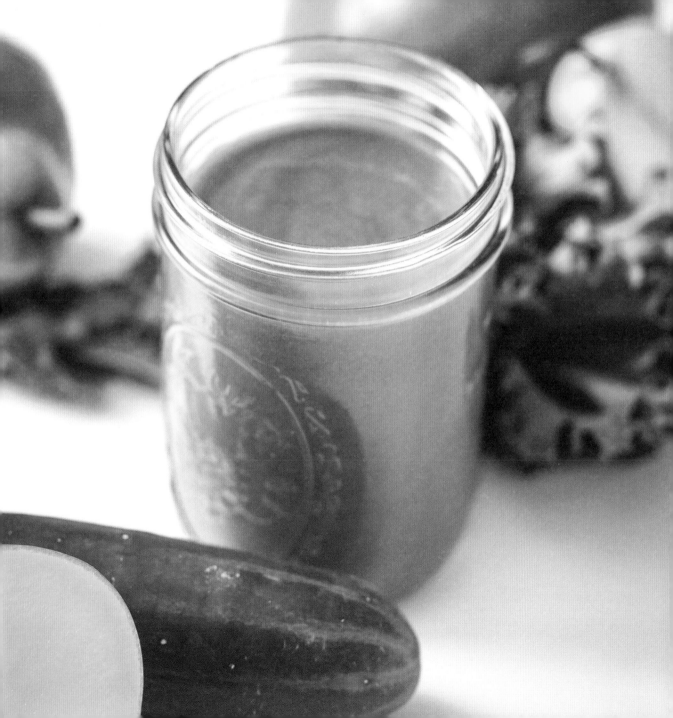

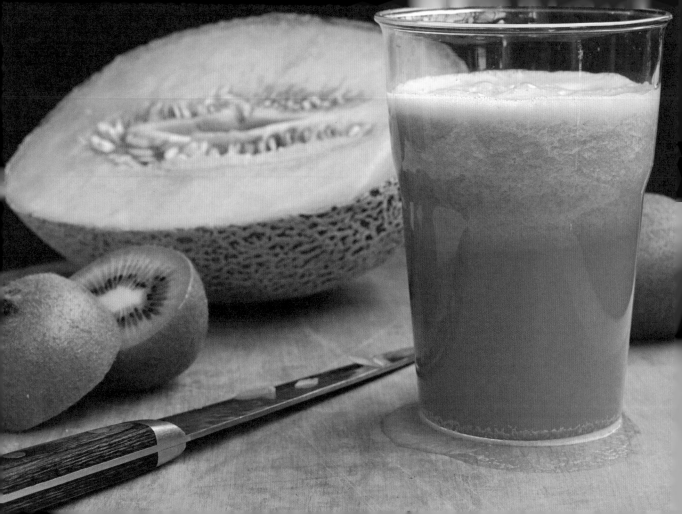

BEAUTY TONIC

½ cucumber

¼ cantaloupe

¼ cup filtered water

1 thumb turmeric

1 teaspoon coconut oil

1 pinch black pepper

Cantaloupe is high in vitamins A and C. I think of it as a beauty fruit, since it nourishes both my skin and hair!

BERRY BLISS

½ cup strawberries (leave the stems on for extra nutrition)

½ cup blueberries

1 ripe banana

½ cup filtered water

½ cup filtered ice

Berries are known for feeding your skin. They have anthocyanin, which is the responsible for their beautiful colors and is a powerful antioxidant. Antioxidants protect your skin from sun damage and protect against the breakdown of your elastin and collagen in your skin.

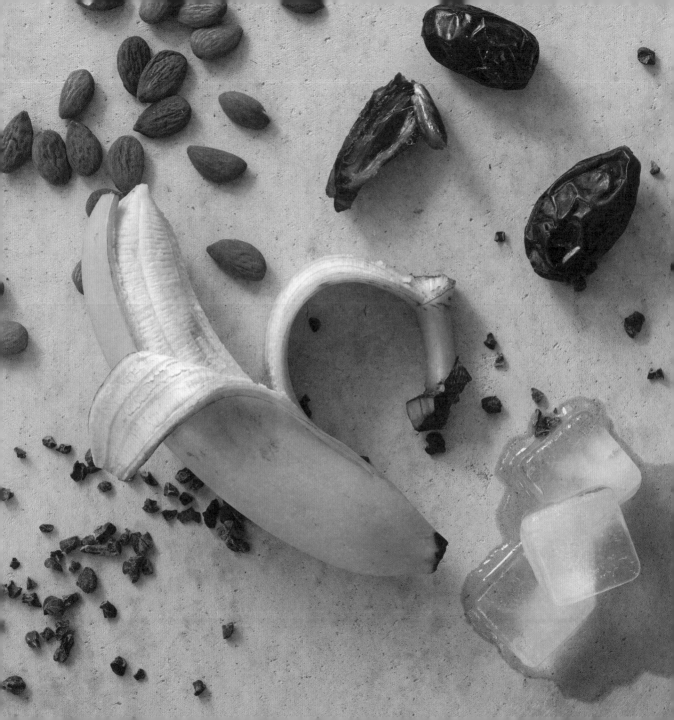

DECADENT SMOOTHIES

The nut milks and seed milks are the base for these, which is why they're more decadent. If you're on a cleanse, I would suggest refraining from having any of these since they're a bit heavier and sweeter. Remember, use the unsweetened version of the milks for these recipes.

APPLE PIE

1 cup almond milk

½ sweet potato

1 tablespoon cinnamon

1 cup ice

½ green apple

Make sure you are using the unsweetened version of the almond milk in this recipe. The sweet potato and green apple will make it sweet enough, even kids will agree.

BIG BANANA

1 cup Brazil nut milk

1 handful mint

½ cup banana

½ date

½ cup ice

½ teaspoon vanilla extract

Trying to get the kids off dairy and sugary ice creams? This is a great place to start! It tastes like dessert, and they won't even know it's good for them. If you want to make it a bit thicker, add more bananas and then they can eat it with a spoon!

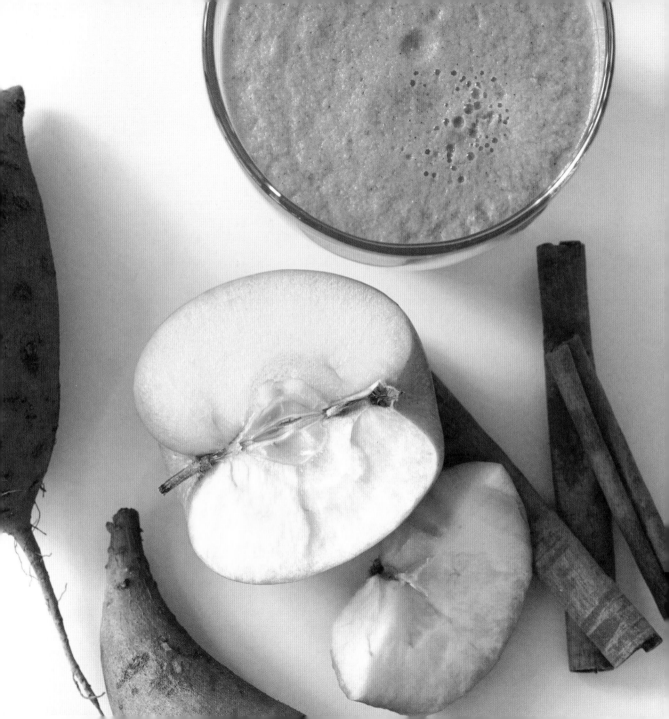

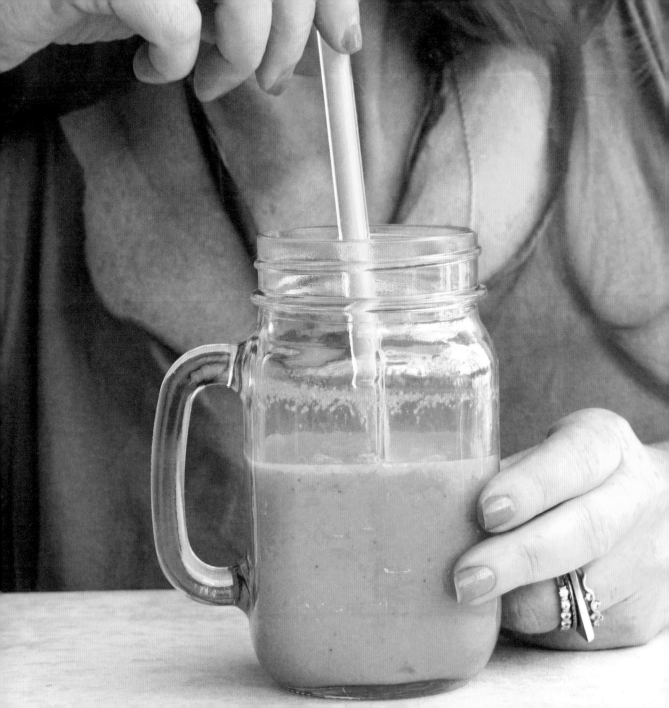

MELON ME

½ cup filtered water

1 cup Brazil nut milk

1 thumb turmeric

½ cup of filtered ice

1 teaspoon coconut oil

⅓ cantaloupe

You might enjoy adding a pinch of cinnamon to this one, which not only makes it taste awesome, but also helps to lower sugar levels!

CHOCOLATE BANANA

1 cup almond milk

1 large tablespoon cacao

½ cup banana

½ cup ice

½ teaspoon vanilla extract

1 pinch salt

Happiness in a glass. This recipe is so good, you will swear it has to be bad for you! Thankfully it is so filled with nutrition, you don't have to feel guilty. The only thing you will feel guilty about is not wanting to share it.

MINT CHOCOLATE CHIP

1 cup almond milk

½ cup ice

½ cup banana

2 oz. cacao nibs

1 large handful mint

2 dates

¼ teaspoon vanilla extract

1 pinch salt

If you would like to make this drink sweeter, I recommend adding dates, coconut palm sugar, lucuma, or honey. Just start with the basics of the recipes that I've listed here and then lightly add more. Just be mindful of how much you are adding so the recipe isn't compromised.

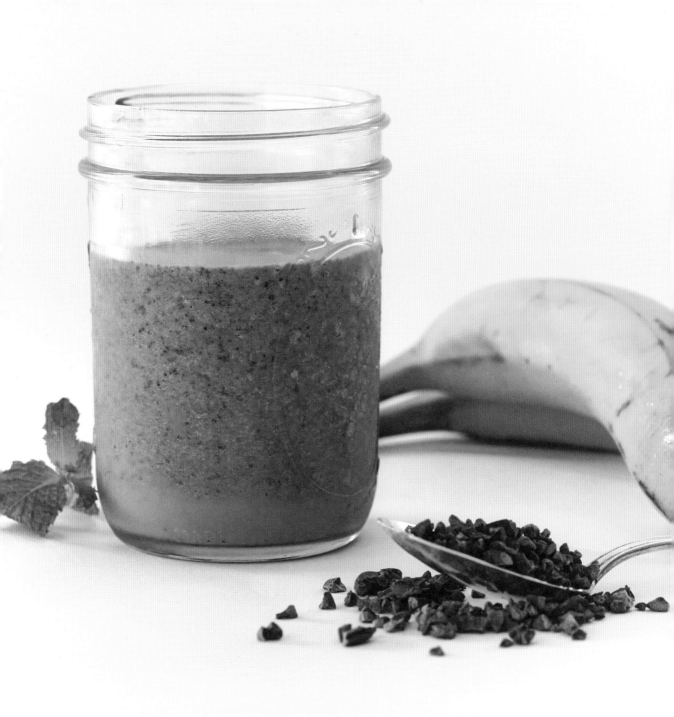

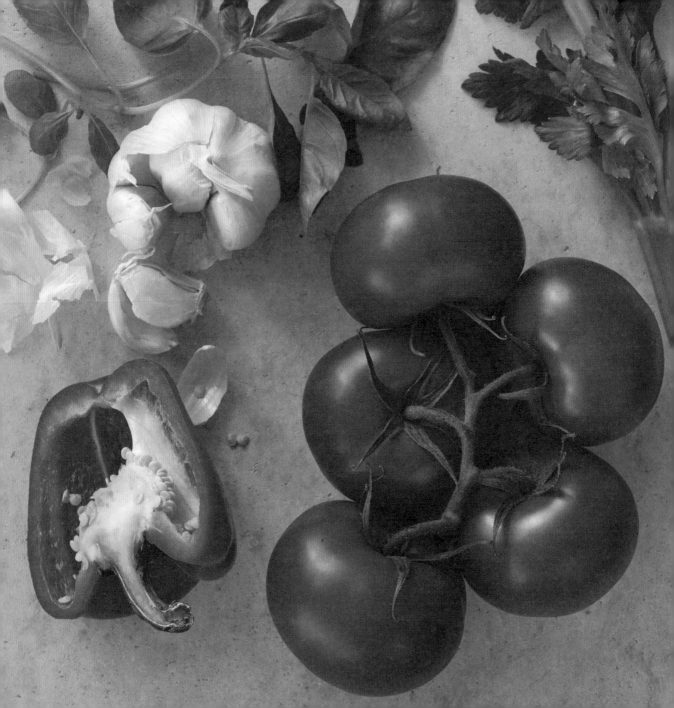

SAVORY SMOOTHIES (A.K.A. SOUPS)

Savory smoothies really fill you up so they are also great while cleansing. These smoothies are also nice to have before dinner as a way of cleansing your palate and helping to ward off unhealthy food choices later on. I love to eat them in a bowl. You can add water if you'd like to thin them out into a drink.

KICKIN' IT GREEN

1 zucchini

1 tomato

2 cloves garlic

1 pinch salt

1 handful cilantro

We often crave the more savory foods on a cleanse, and this is a great way to get it in. If you don't love garlic, start with 1 clove and see if you need to add another.

RED & GREEN

¼ onion

1 tomato

1 handful cilantro

4 stalks celery

¼ red bell pepper

If you want to take this recipe up a notch, add a small bit of olive oil or avocado, or maybe even a little cayenne pepper. Add your own touch! Just be mindful that if you are on a cleanse—go light with the oils and avocado.

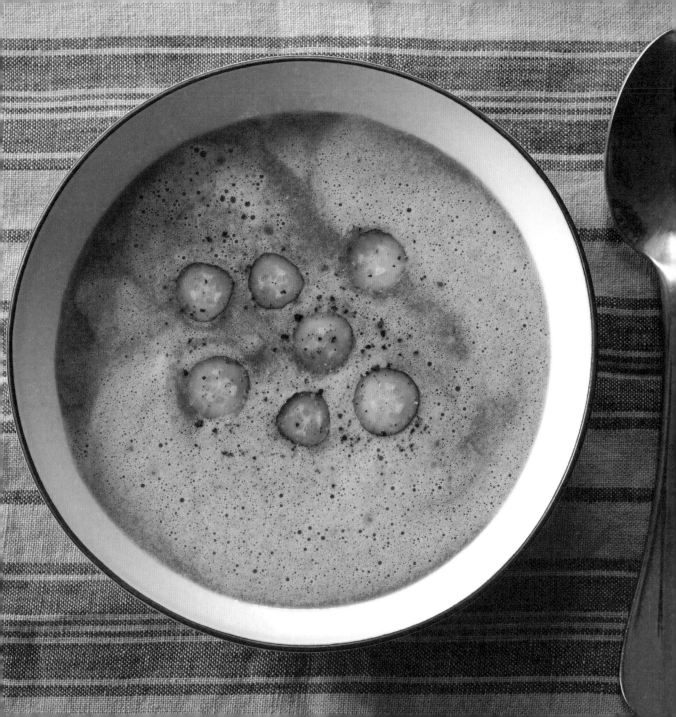

AVOCADO KICK

3 kale leaves

¼ avocado

4 basil leaves

1 handful cilantro

1 large pinch salt

1 teaspoon olive oil

2 tomatoes

1 cucumber

2 cloves garlic

Avocado, quite possibly my favorite food on the planet, is a great source of fat. What I also love about avocado is its ability to change the texture of your smoothie or soup. It makes them thicker and heartier. If you are looking to be more "filled up," avocado is a great ingredient to add to both your savory soups and sweet smoothies.

LIGHT LOVE

3 chard leaves

¼ avocado

1 handful cilantro

½ cup water

½ zucchini

1 pinch salt

This is a delicate green soup and is quite light. If you want it a bit heavier, add more of the avocado. Keep plenty of water in it, as it helps it to blend better. With some recipes, we need more liquid to get the blender moving. I often add water to make this happen. Go slow with the water; this way you keep the taste but it helps the blender blades move.

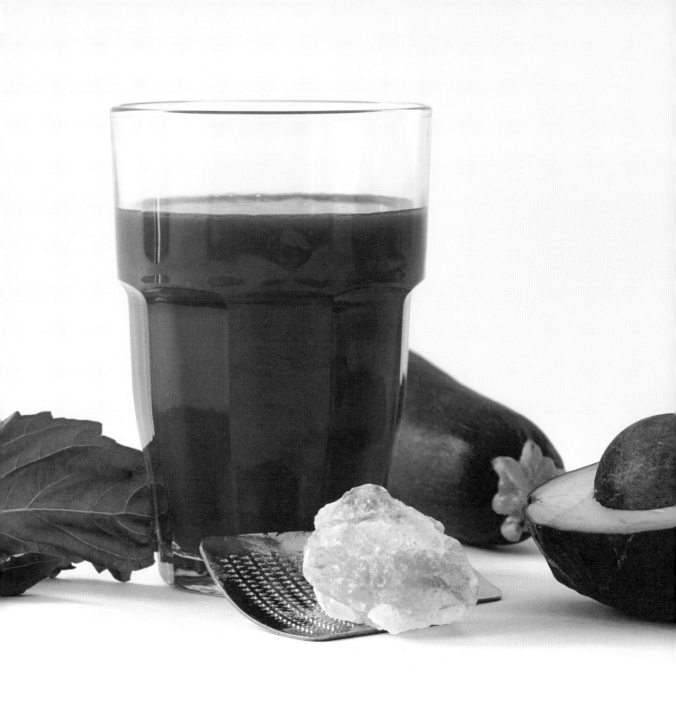

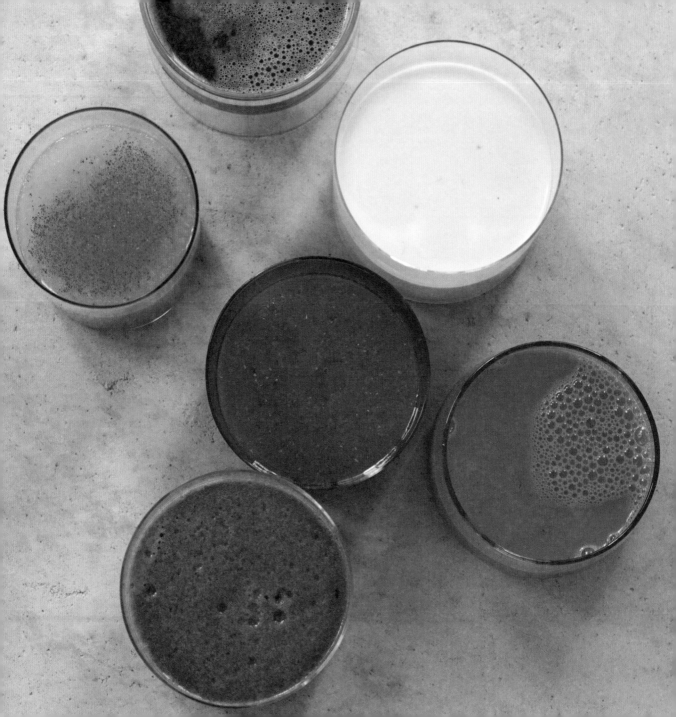

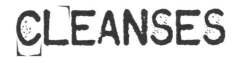

CLEANSES

What Is a Cleanse?

"The doctor of the future will give no medicine, but will interest her or his patients in the care of the human frame, in a proper diet, and in the cause and prevention of disease."—Thomas A. Edison

Cleansing is quite the buzzword these days. So, what is it really about? And who should do it? A cleanse is simply about giving your body a break. It's a chance for your body to work a bit less than it does every day. There are varying degrees of cleansing. For some, switching one day from a cooked meal to an organic, raw, fresh smoothie is a cleanse. For others, staying on liquids for a week is detoxing. What's best for you depends on what your starting point is and what you are looking to gain.

When cleansing, we benefit not just on a physical level, but also on spiritual one. It is a time to go deep inside yourself and clear your mind and head space. Let go of the distractions. Rest and re-energize. Again, just switching out your morning bagel for a green smoothie with fruit is a great step in the right direction.

There is an idea in the health arena called crowding out. It does not necessarily mean leaving things out, but instead advocates that the more nourishing and real food you put into your body, the less room and desire you have to fill it with junk food. When you start to pay attention to how you feel after you eat, you often start to make healthier choices.

Ideally, I recommend a three to five day cleanse to start. During the cleansing process, you have to pay attention to your body. Pay attention to if you are actually hungry or whether you might be bored or anxious. When you are cleansing, it is a great time to examine your habits around food because we often eat for reasons other than actual hunger.

WHO WE ARE

We are a Raw, Vegan, Organic, Gluten Free cafe that also offers delivery, take out and a full line of Cleanse options. Our drinks & dishes are abundant in flavor and contain no animal products, grains, gluten, fillers or preservatives of any kind. Find out more at gingersnapsorganic.com

GINGERSNAPSORGANIC.COM • 130 EAST 7TH ST. NYC.

[GO] Beet

[GINGERSNAP'S ORGANIC]
cafe & specialty cleanses

RAW • VEGAN • GLUTEN-FREE

shake well

Ingredients:

"All Organic, Cold Pressed, Unpasteurized"

Beets, Carrots, Pear, Ginger

NET CONTENTS 17 FL OZ

WHO WE ARE

We are a Raw, Vegan, Organic, Gluten Free cafe that also offers delivery, take out and a full line of Cleanse options. Our drinks & dishes are abundant in flavor and contain no animal products, grains, gluten, fillers or preservatives of any kind. Find out more at gingersnapsorganic.com

SNAPSORGANIC.COM • 130 EAST 7TH ST. NYC.

[GO] Heat

[GINGERSNAP'S ORGANIC]
cafe & specialty cleanses

RAW • VEGAN • GLUTEN-FREE

shake well

Ingredients:

"All Organic, Cold Pressed, Unpasteurized"

Orange, Ginger, Tumeric, Cayenne

NET CONTENTS 17 FL OZ

WHO WE ARE

We are a Raw, Vegan, Organic, Gluten Free cafe that also offers delivery, take out and a full line of Cleanse options. Our drinks & dishes are abundant in flavor and contain no animal products, grains, gluten, fillers or preservatives of any kind. Find out more at gingersnapsorganic.com

GINGERSNAPSORGANIC.COM • 130 EAST 7TH ST. NYC.

[GO] Vanilla Superfood Milk

[GINGERSNAP'S ORGANIC]
cafe & specialty cleanses

shake well

Ingredients:

"All Organic, Cold Pressed, Unpasteurized"

Almond Milk (Raw Unpasteurized Almonds, Filtered Water), Vanilla

NET CONTENTS 17 FL OZ

☞ 10 RULES FOR CLEANSES

1. Have at least six drinks a day (more if you are very active) but I do not recommend less, even if you do not feel hungry. Remember, we are trying to rest the body, not starve it.
2. Drink half your weight in ounces of water a day.
3. A juice takes about thirty minutes to digest, so wait at least that amount of time before you go on to the next.
4. Smoothies and nut milks take about an hour to digest, so wait at least that amount of time before you go on to the next.
5. Let the drinks sit in your mouth so they can start to digest there. Your mouth is the key to digestion.
6. Do use mindfulness when drinking them—do not just gulp any of them down.
7. Try to start your first drink within an hour of rising and the last within four hours of sleeping. Again this is ideal, but not a must.
8. Do your best to stick to the plan. It is easy to get frustrated and completely toss in the towel, but don't do that. If you slip up, forgive yourself and then just get back on your cleanse.
9. If you are active, add a vegan, grain-free, plant-based organic protein powder to your nut milk.
10. Be good to yourself!

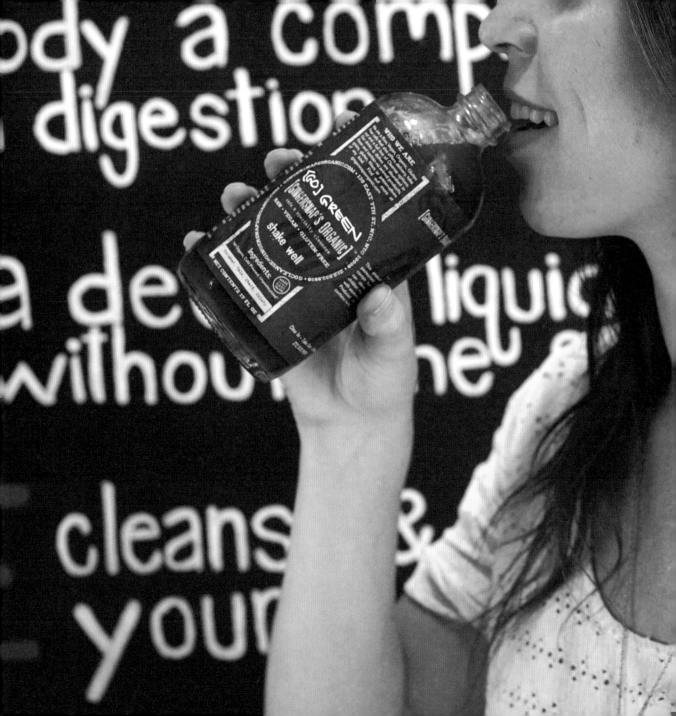

Why It's Important To Cleanse

"What you do today can improve all your tomorrows."—Ralph Marston

Dangerous toxins can gather in your body and, if they're not properly eliminated, they can compromise the immune system and manifest as a variety of health conditions. Going on a cleanse is a great way to give your body a break and put it into high gear for a fresh start.

When It's Time To Cleanse

Some signs it's time for a cleanse: constipation, gas, bloating, headaches, joint pain, sluggishness, irritability, skin problems, and bad breath. The change of seasons is a nice natural point to use to begin a cleanse, or if you feel you are in a rut and your energy is sluggish.

What To Expect When You Start Your Cleanse

For some people, they instantly feel energized and amazing; for others, it might be a bit more difficult at first. Sometimes, for the first few days, your body might resist the fresh start you're bringing it and this might include experiencing some headaches, dizziness, nausea, fatigue, skin eruptions, and constipation. If these symptoms persist, it is important to stop the cleanse and consult with a doctor. It is common to feel hungry for the first one to two days. When you feel hungry, first try water. If after that you still feel you really *need* something, add an additional drink to the cleanse. You must pay attention to your body. If you are really feeling bad, add more drinks to your cleanse. I suggest starting with six, but for you eight might be a better number. You have to pay attention to your body!

What Can I Eat?

The recipes in the book are great for cleansing. I have laid out the recipes into different categories. You will notice there are different levels of cleanses in this section that have you eat different things—look through them and choose what is right for you. If you are going to add food, it should be raw, organic fruits and vegetables.

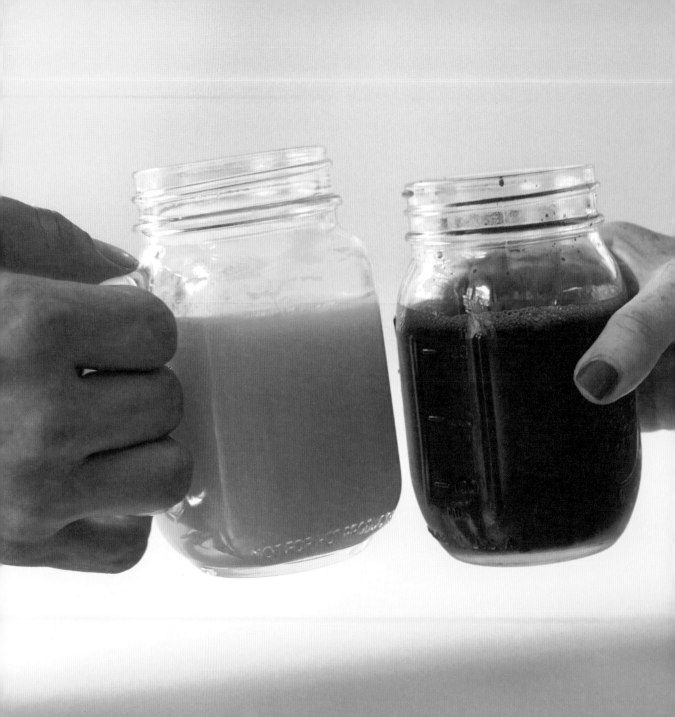

Which Cleanse Should I Choose?

"You must know that in any moment a decision you make can change the course of your life forever."—Tony Robbins

As you see, the recipes are laid out into different sections so depending on what level you're cleansing at, you will choose drinks from different chapters. Below are all the different levels of cleansing. I usually recommend one- to five-day cleanses depending on where you're at, but please consult your doctor before beginning and pay attention to your body. If you want to go longer on the cleanse, you can go longer. If you're feeling ill, stop or add in more drinks.

Level 1

You are new to cleansing. The thought of drinking something green is scary, and you don't want to do it! If this is you, my suggestion would be to start with:

- Detox Juice (start your day with this—as soon as you wake up)
- Green Juice with Fruit or Citrus Fruit (have about a half hour after the detox juice)
- Fruit Smoothie
- Flavored Nut Milk

- Savory Smoothie (a.k.a. soup)
- Green Fruit Smoothie (choose one that has greens in it)

Level 2

If you always start your day with a green juice and eat healthy, but you've never cleansed before, these are the right drinks for you!

- Detox Juice (start your day with this—as soon as you wake up)
- All Green Juice (have about a half hour after the detox juice)
- Green Juice with Fruit or Citrus Fruit
- Flavored Nut Milk
- Savory Smoothie
- Green Fruit Smoothie (choose one with greens in it)

Level 3

You have cleansed before and you want to take it to the next level.

- Detox Juice (start your day with this—as soon as you wake up)
- All Green Juice (have about a half hour after the detox juice)
- Green Juice with Fruit or Citrus Fruit
- Savory Smoothie
- All Green Juice
- Nut Milk (sweetened or unsweetened)

Level 4

You want to cleanse, but you want to keep your fiber! This cleanse uses mostly blended smoothies and stays away from the juices. In doing this, you keep the fiber in!

- Detox Juice (start your day with this—as soon as you wake up)
- Green Fruit Smoothie
- Savory Smoothie (a.k.a. soup)
- Green Fruit Smoothie
- Savory Smoothie (a.k.a. soup)
- Nut Milk (sweetened or unsweetened)

Level 5

I want to leave out all the sugar!

- Detox Juice (start your day with this—as soon as you wake up)
- All Green Juice
- Savory Juice (a.k.a. soup)
- All Green Juice
- Savory Smoothie (a.k.a. soup)
- Nut Milk (unsweetened)

As you can see, there are many ways to mix and match your cleansing plan, depending on where you are at and what you are looking to accomplish! What's most important is to play and pay attention. See how you feel in your body! Have fun!

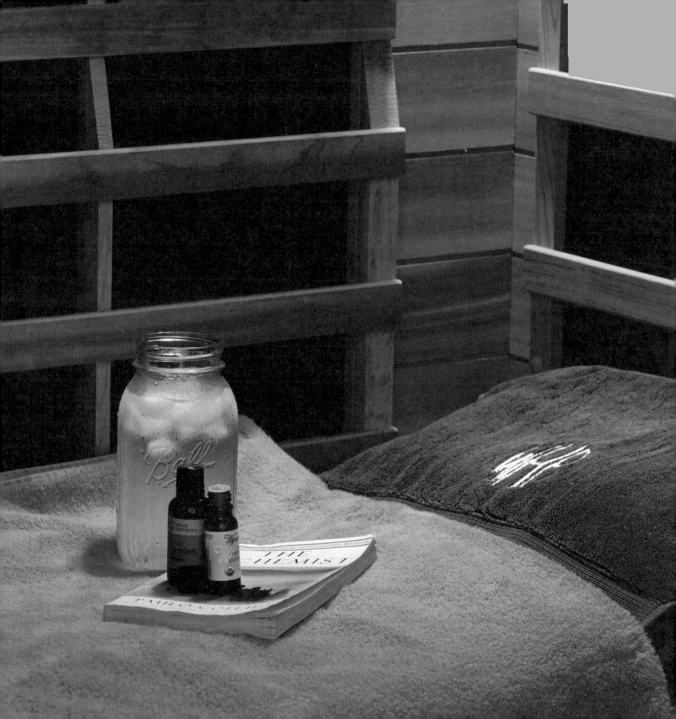

Deeper Cleansing

Saunas and Infrared Saunas

Sweating is good for you. A sauna detox helps you sweat out toxins and aids in anti-aging, pain relief, improved circulation, and overall cell health. It's the body's safest and most natural way to heal and maintain good health. An infrared sauna is a type of sauna that uses light to create heat. These saunas are sometimes called far-infrared saunas, where the infrared waves fall on the light spectrum. A traditional sauna uses heat to warm the air, which in turn warms your body. An infrared sauna heats your body directly without warming the air around you. The appeal of saunas in general is that they cause reactions, such as vigorous sweating and increased heart rate, similar to those elicited by moderate exercise. An infrared sauna produces these results at lower temperatures than does a regular sauna, which makes it accessible to people who can't tolerate the heat of a conventional sauna.

Meditation

Meditation is a very personal experience for everyone. More and more research supports the idea that meditation is the key to living every day from the perspective of grateful mindfulness. If you're new to meditation, I suggest first working with a guided meditation. Many can be found online. Even playing calming music is a great start to closing your eyes and quieting your mind.

Yoga

It's important to bring yoga into every exercise routine and it's especially nice to do when you're on a cleanse. Because of the deep breathing, the slowing down, the turns and twists of your upper body in the practice, it's another tool to help twist out your organs. It's also about bringing the healing energy of breath into your practice. Prana Yama is a great option for cleansing and rejuvenating your organs through breathing. I suggest opting for the meditative version of a yoga class where you're able to do a lot of breath work.

Some of my favorites are hot yoga, yin yoga, kundalini—the best would be a yoga that's more meditative and not a vinyasa music flow class. Regardless of whether you're going to a class or finding a session online, I'd suggest a slow, mindful practice that allows you to go inward while you're cleansing.

Dry Brush Massage

A dry brush is a great way to enhance detoxification and cleanse the pores. Use the brush from head to toe, always moving it in a small circular motion over your skin. Follow this with a hot and cold shower combination. This is great for stimulating the lymphatic system, increasing circulation, and removing dead skin cells!

Tongue Scraping

Scraping the tongue daily removes any build-up on the tongue, which, if left untreated, can lead to bad breath and a build up of bacteria. By removing this coating, you also improve your ability to taste your food, which makes it more satisfying. By increasing your taste reception, not only do you eat less, you also eliminate the need to add more sugar, salt, or excessive spice to the food to make it more flavorful.

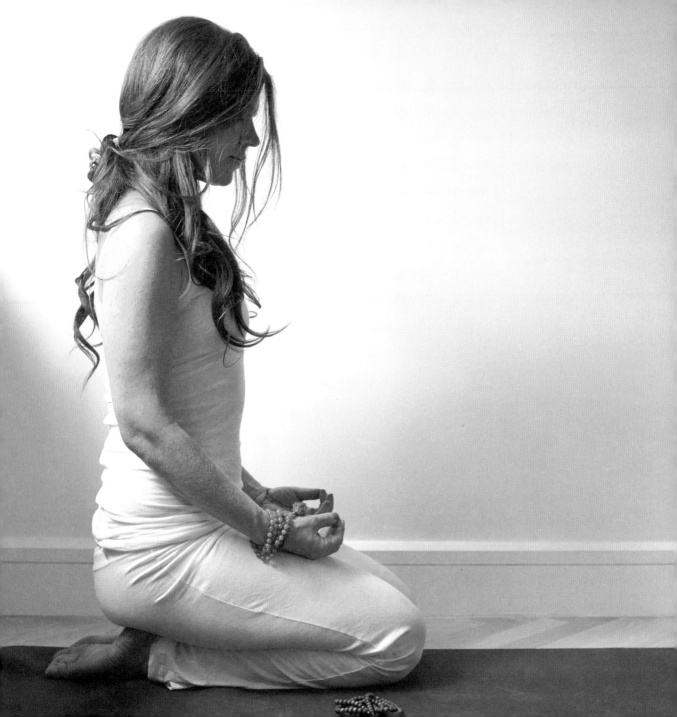

Let's Sum It Up!

We've made it to the end of this journey, but it's also the beginning of a fresh way of looking at all that fruits and vegetables can do for you. It's about balance and about making the best choices we can make every day for what foods to put in our bodies. It doesn't have to be difficult, or require a lot of work, but adding juices and smoothies is a great way to start experimenting with all the goodness nature offers. Take it a step at a time, and a day at a time, and I hope you'll see that small steps of adding more fruits and vegetables to your life will start to lift you up into the healthier and more energized way of living that you've been searching for.

And, if you're ever in New York City, stop by Gingersnap's Organic to say hi!

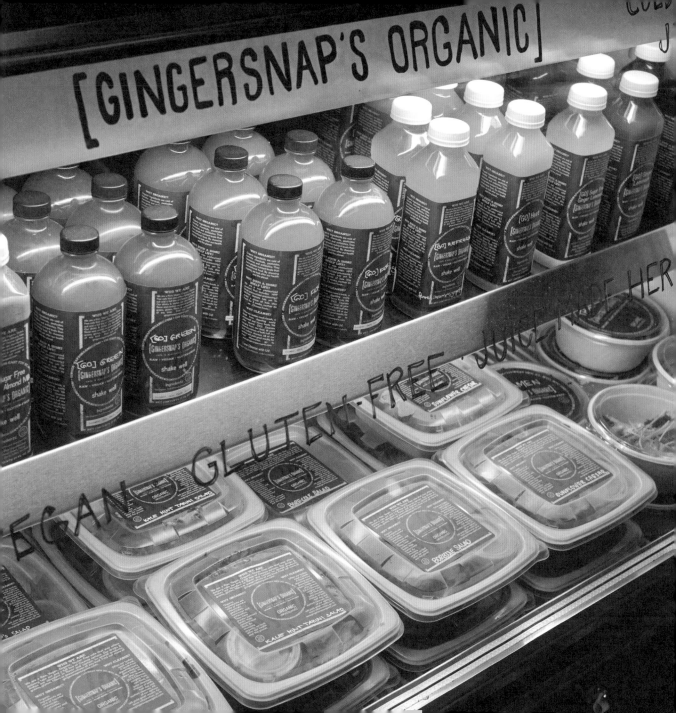